Praise f[...]

"Brilliant… This book holds [...] quality of life when living with osteoporosis. [...] own experience, lessons learned, and extensive research, Christine Thomas has created the most valuable tool/resource to help women like me rebuild their lives after suffering from osteoporosis."

- Norma Vernon, osteoporosis patient, British Columbia

"For several years Christine has researched how to build better bones and regain life after spinal fracture. Her indomitable spirit shines through everything she does and provides hope and encouragement to the many women who are reaching out to live well with osteoporosis."

- Dr. Susan Fisher, MD, CCFP, FCFP

"*Unbreakable* speaks to any woman who wants to make a change for the better. Christine's candid story will empower you to become an effective advocate on your own behalf, and may even inspire you to help others living with osteoporosis."

- Ryan Clarke, LL.B., President, Advocacy Solutions

"A powerful book… an excellent resource for women searching for straightforward steps to improve their bone health."

- Peggy McColl, New York Times best-selling author

"An amazing, compelling and informative must read for all women who care about their bone health. Christine Thomas provides excellent insight into living well with osteoporosis. She is passionate about educating people about the need to take care of their bones and through her actions she provides hope, enc[...] inspiration to all."

- Angela Haines-Wangda, MSc. Rehab, BSc PT, MCPA, D.O. (

Praise for Unbreakable

"I have known Christine through her journey back to good health. I admire her amazing spirit and strength as she has successfully reclaimed back her life from debilitating osteoporotic fractures; recreating a great life, that allows her to take care of herself and of her young family—and sharing with all of us her hope that yes, what you do can change your life for the better.

Christine is a role model to all of us—she walked her talk, and I am fortunate to have met and worked with her on her journey back to health and quality of life. Christine shares with us what works and how she made it back—an amazing journey and inspiring story."

- Catherine Morisset, Life Wellness Coach

"Christine Thomas is a tireless champion in the battle against osteoporosis. *Unbreakable,* the remarkable story of Christine's triumph over adversity, is sure to bring hope and inspiration to women struggling with osteoporosis."

- Elizabeth Contestabile RN, BScN, NCMP, Nurse Educator,
Shirley E. Greenberg Women's Health Centre

UNBREAKABLE:

A WOMAN'S TRIUMPH OVER OSTEOPOROSIS

BY CHRISTINE THOMAS

Published by Partner Publishing, Ottawa, Canada

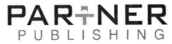

www.partnerpublishing.com

Cover design by Donald Lanouette (design@partnerpublishing.com)

Disclaimer: While the author and publisher have made reasonable effort to ensure that all information in this book is accurate as of October 2010, it is not in any fashion intended to replace the advice and care of medical professionals. Neither the publishers nor the author are engaged in rendering professional advice or services to the individual reader. All matters regarding your health require medical supervision. Neither the author nor the publishers shall be liable or responsible for any loss, injury, or damage allegedly arising from any information or suggestion in this book. If you suspect that you have bone health issues it is important to see your doctor.

Unbreakable: A Woman's Triumph over Osteoporosis
Christine Thomas
www.christinethomas.com

Includes bibliographical references and resource contacts

ISBN: 9780978470135

1. Osteoporosis –a patient's perspective
2. Health / Wellness / Fitness

To Gerry and Chanel,
thank you for your love and
support throughout this journey.

You are the reason I am *Unbreakable*.

TABLE OF CONTENTS

Table of Contents

Table of Contents

Chapter 17
Knowledge is Power: Making Sense of Medications
& Alternative Treatments 215

Table of Contents

With Thanks and Appreciation

My heartfelt thanks to:

Cherrie Fergusson, for her incredible ability to put the right word in the right place and her unfailing encouragement for me to tell my story.

The exceptionally skilled and talented team of Partner Publishing: Donald Lanouette, for being such a great listener and for his patience and creativity; his designs made this book come alive; Karen Opas, Editor extraordinaire, for her highly-skilled editing and for her enthusiasm, humour, and commitment to ensure this book made it to print. You are amazing!

Peggy McColl, for her kindness, helping me stay on track, and keeping me motivated. Your enthusiasm is contagious!

Marq Nelson, Sabrina Paiva, Vicky Johnston, and Denise Deby for taking time out of their hectic schedules to provide input when I needed it, which made this book an even better resource for people wanting to improve their bone health.

The staff and volunteers of Osteoporosis Canada, especially Anita Nevins, who answered my first call for help in my darker days and Ann Bortolotti whose endless determination helped a chapter grow and thrive in Canada's capital.

My past and present bone health team: Dr. John Gay, Dr. Ann Cranney, Dr. Susan Fisher, Dr. Susan Humprey-Murto, Dr. Leeanne Ward, Dr. Sarah Nikkel, Dr. Elaine Jolly, Dr. Jordan Pettigrew, Jennifer Roberts-Teale and Lori Garlough (dental hygienists), Elizabeth Contestabile (Nurse Educator), Angela Wangda (osteopathic manual practitioner), Catherine Morisset (life wellness coach), Adoracion de leon and Doracelia Bautista (care-givers), Diane Craig (image consultant), Anne-Marie Tessier (hair stylist), and Pat Armstrong (esthetician), for your knowledge, skills, compassion, encouragement and endless patience in answering my questions! Without their help and guidance I would not be living well with osteoporosis.

To my parents, for their love and support. I began writing this book when my mother and father—Helen and Ed Thomas—were alive. Sadly, they are not here to read it. To my family and extended family, especially Judy Latremoille, Susan Merkley, Lynne MacMillan, Patricia Brown, and Lisa Chartier-Derouin. Thank you for being there when I needed you most. You're the best!

My dear friends Fiona Potter, Peggy MacPhail, Christine Lamothe, Kathleen Bradley, Brenda Whitten, Joanne Evans, and Patti Magee, for your suggestions, feedback, and encouragement throughout my stages of building better bones and this book. And to all the "alumni parents" of Westboro Village Cooperative pre-school and the parents of Chanel's Elmdale schoolmates, thank you for your incredible support.

Writing this book meant many personal sacrifices for my family. I want to thank my husband Gerry and my daughter Chanel for their love and support throughout the journey of writing this book, for encouraging me to realize my dream of publishing this book, and for never doubting my ability to complete it. Mommy can now come out of the computer room and play!

FOREWORD

I met Christine Thomas when I was president of Osteoporosis Canada and she agreed to share her personal journey as a spokeswoman in order to help other women become aware that, even in their 30's, they might be at risk for osteoporosis. Christine had just given birth to her first child when, bending over the crib of her infant daughter, she fractured her spine. Like many who are diagnosed with osteoporosis, she had assumed it was a disease of old age and that her healthy lifestyle would protect her.

Unbreakable shares all the hard-won knowledge, both practical and emotional, that Christine gained as she fought the long battle of recovery from her fractures and prevention of future breaks. This book differs from any other book on bone health. It will give you the knowledge and support required to journey towards the healthiest bones possible, both before and after fracture.

Read her story and imagine what it must have felt like to receive the devastating news that she could **never, ever** bend over to pick up her daughter again. As a mother (and now grandmother), I can't imagine the horror of knowing that each time my child cried, it would have to be someone else who picked her up to hand her to me—or she would be left to cry without my comforting embrace. Close your eyes and imagine what that would be like.

From the moment I met Christine I found her courageous and generous. She has faced this disease head-on and now she is sharing her experience in how we can take care of our bones, no matter our age. She stresses the importance of being your own health advocate. She has already made a difference in many lives because of her amazing volunteer efforts with Osteoporosis Canada.

Now she is sharing the information she gathered in her quest to regain her health and, perhaps even more important to someone facing the same struggle, the insights she gained in how to deal with pain, injury, medication, the health system and stay motivated while fighting through it to better bone health.

With sheer determination, Christine began a journey of recovery that has allowed her to reclaim her life. Christine is living proof that bone loss and fracture can happen to anyone at any age. She also proves that, whether pre or post fracture, there are always steps that can be taken towards improving bone health and quality of life.

- Karen Ormerod, former President & CEO, Osteoporosis Canada

INTRODUCTION

I was 42 when Osteoporosis left me with the weakened and brittle bones of a 90-year-old. Unfortunately, I was unaware of this until an event that changed the course of my life forever. As I bent over my newborn daughter's crib, a jolting pain shot through my spine, nearly causing me to pass out. Luckily, my husband was nearby to catch me from falling. The next day, my physician prescribed pain medication for a muscle spasm and sent me home.

Although I continued to experience daily back pain, I accepted it as a side effect of my recent pregnancy and hoped it would eventually go away. My medications didn't relieve the pain enough to prevent me from spending most of my time in bed, the only place where I could find some relief from the nightmare I was living.

The pain continued, along with visits to the hospital, for several more weeks until physicians finally identified the cause of my pain from a bone scan that confirmed I was suffering from five fractures to my spine caused by a disease I would later learn is called "The Silent Disease," osteoporosis. I was diagnosed with a severe case of it. So severe that just the simple act of bending over to lift my daughter from her crib had caused the fractures.

Like the estimated 100 million other women worldwide whose bodies are silently suffering from bone disease, it was too late to stop the crippling side-effects from occurring by the time I learned of my sickness. After weeks of trips to and from hospitals and doctors' offices, I grew impatient for results; I wanted my former life back— the one without constant pain and with the freedom of mobility.

Following the diagnosis, I began a treatment program that included appointments with physicians, physiotherapists, occupational therapists, and an endocrinologist. Although they provided me with the best medical care, I realized there would never be one "Doctor of Osteoporosis" who could bundle and treat all my physical and emotional care needs. And regardless of their individual concerns, there was so little time that they could spend with me during the appointment. It was then that I decided that if I truly wanted to get back to life, I would have to do it myself.

Years later, after thousands of hours researching osteoporosis and fracture, hundreds of trips to hospitals, physicians' offices, and physiotherapists, and countless conversations with the wonderful staff and volunteers I worked with as chair of the Ottawa Chapter of Osteoporosis Canada (OCOC), I discovered that there is hope, even for those of us who are diagnosed after the shock of suffering the crippling side effects of fracture. It's not too late to get back much of what was lost, and it's not too late to help the millions of women worldwide who, unbeknown to them, are silently losing bone mass that could eventually lead to the disease and broken bones.

My journey begins in the throes of pain, suffering, tears, and the depression that soon enveloped me, and ends with the new life I fought so hard to get. It's a journey of learning, coping, tolerance, and a powerful knowledge that empowers, motivates, and drives me to live life to the fullest, every day. I share my story so that other woman can get their lives back, too.

As proceeds from sales of this book go to Osteoporosis Canada, your purchase is both an investment in your bone health and the bone health of all Canadians.

Note to the Reader

This book is my story and it includes my opinions as well as extensive evidence-based research. It is meant to help prepare you for your appointments with your doctor and other members of your health care team. This book is not a substitute for the advice of your physician or health-care provider. Each of you is unique and so is your medical history. Before attempting any exercises or implementing any changes suggested in this book, you must discuss them with your physician.

CHAPTER 1

~

CHANGES & HOPE: WHAT TO EXPECT WITH A FRACTURE DIAGNOSIS

My spinal fractures changed my life—at times it felt like they had taken it away from me. I have regained my life and the ability to enjoy it, but I had no idea of the tough journey I was about to embark on. I spent a lot time in pain. I spent a lot of time angry at myself—for not paying more attention to my bone health—and angry at my doctors—for not having diagnosed my osteoporosis before fracture. Once the problem was discovered, I spent a lot of time in the offices of various health professionals. Initially, it felt like my life was an unending round of pain and medical appointments. I needed to become an active participant in reclaiming my life. The health professionals who helped me were wonderful people, but I was the person with the biggest stake in my bone health.

Desperate to manage the disease that was keeping me practically bedridden, I spent endless hours researching osteoporosis and fracture from osteoporosis. It was a difficult and often exhausting job to gather accurate information. I wanted to make educated decisions about managing osteoporosis and, in particular, controlling the painful and emotional side effects from the fractures which were my first crushing indicator (and the brutal consequence of living with osteoporosis for years without knowing it).

During my journey to recovery I discovered two key findings:

1. Osteoporosis can strike at any age.
2. In the majority of cases it goes undetected even after fracture.

1

It remains under-diagnosed and under-treated by medical professionals, even in high-risk patients.

The result is a complacent expectation in our society that weakened bones, especially in women, are a routine complication of aging that we are destined to live with. Although there have been several significant scientific advances in osteoporosis research in recent years, the information is largely lost along the way somewhere during the trickle down effect from research lab to physician to patient. Undiagnosed, the rate of life-altering fracture in women and men is proportionally higher than what it could be with an earlier diagnosis.

I also discovered how widespread this disease has become. Globally, osteoporosis affects more than 200 million women and men. The incidence of osteoporosis is nearly as common as high blood pressure and more common than high cholesterol. The statistics show that worldwide, one in three women and one in five men over 50 years of age will suffer in their lifetime at least one fracture by osteoporosis. As I have learned from my own experience, the life changes from fracture can be devastating, turning an active life into one of pain, disability, and dependence.

A good denotation for osteoporosis is the "3D" disease, with the three "Ds" standing for devastating, debilitating, and depressing. Devastating, because the disease is progressive and cannot be cured. Potentially debilitating when there is fracture, particularly in the spine or hip. Depressing because of alterations in physique, posture, and mobility that result in a quality of life change for the worse. The physical and emotional changes which cause the most significant life alterations are:

- Increased difficulty in performing activities in daily life

- Chronic pain

- Loss of height, muscle tone, and the ability to stand, walk, or both

- Decreased body strength and limitations on physical capacity

- Permanent physical deformity such as a kyphosis or "hunchback"

- Crowding of internal organs

- Prolonged or permanent disability

- Fear, anxiety, depression, and other emotional pain.

Over time, these life changes become overwhelming, leading to more serious, long-lasting life changes:

- Low self-esteem

- Loss of income

- Negative impact on family life

- Loss of independence, and in some cases, complete dependence on others.

Weak bones affect all women and men in one way or another. In addition to loss of physical, emotional, and financial well-being, the cost to the health care system for treating osteoporosis is staggering. According to the International Osteoporosis Foundation, in 2005 there were more than 2 million osteoporotic fractures within North America alone, costing an estimated $19 billion. Without effective prevention and treatment strategies, by 2025 costs in North America could soar to more than $25 billion for treating osteoporotic fractures.

Your bone health is determined by what you are doing right now to keep your bones as strong and healthy as possible—it's never too early or too late to begin a strong bone health plan. The bad news is that no matter your age or risk factors, you will always be susceptible to osteoporosis and fracture as you age. There is hope, however. Osteoporosis can be controlled and its fractures prevented through treatment, diet, and exercise. Yet because of its invisible symptoms, paired with certain myths and misconceptions about the disease, osteoporosis continues to take its toll on men and women alike.

CHAPTER 2

~

"MYTH" CONCEPTIONS ABOUT OSTEOPOROSIS

We tend to take our bones for granted, perhaps even think of them as unchanging, more akin to rock than to our supple skin. In fact, bones are made up of living cells and are constantly in the process of construction and demolition. When this cycle becomes unbalanced, bones can weaken and become brittle, more like glass than stone. There is rarely any pain (until it is too late). We can't look in the mirror and see our bones. And the medical tests are nowhere near as simple as for other common medical conditions like diabetes or high blood pressure.

If we do think about osteoporosis, we slot it in as a disease of extreme old age and malnourishment. We don't apply it to ourselves. We believe the myths and misinformation that I also believed—until I was slapped into reality by spinal fractures.

One of my bone health mentors, life wellness coach Catherine Morisset, realized early in her career that many of her clients misunderstood or were misinformed about bone disease. Osteoporosis was rampant in her family—her grandmother's osteoposis led to not one but two broken hips, which probably explains why she exudes an incredible passion for helping women and men improve their bone health. She wants everyone to be aware of the simple physical and nutritional changes that could not only stop osteoporosis' progression, but even restore bone loss in many cases. She has identified the top nine common myths that most significantly impact the bone health of her clients.

Myth No.1: Only the Elderly Get Osteoporosis

Although osteoporosis is a condition most commonly experienced by men and women over 50 years, it is also found in younger adults.

Women especially are at greater risk than men because of increased bone mass loss after menopause. Because osteoporosis is a silent disease that has no symptoms, women as young as their early 40s are shocked to learn their bones are losing density at a rapid rate and can be well on their way to fragility, the precursor to debilitating fractures. What they want to avoid is loss of bone that is so significant that their bones become thin, brittle, and fragile like mine, to the point of breaking at the slightest bump or jolt. Being diagnosed with severe osteoporosis and five spinal fractures at the age of 42 indicates the onset of osteoporosis for me probably began as early as my 30's.

Myth No. 2: You Won't Get Osteoporosis If You Eat a Balanced Diet, Drink Plenty of Milk, & Take Calcium Supplements

To keep our bones healthy, it is well publicized that our bodies require bone-building nutrition like calcium, and vitamin D with the calcium to help absorb it.

Calcium and vitamin D must be combined with another crucial element, physical activity, to be the most effective. Maintaining healthy bones requires attention to basic elements that are the building blocks of good health and strong bones. This is especially true for postmenopausal women. Studies have shown that bone density in postmenopausal women can be maintained or increased with a combination of adequate levels of calcium and vitamin D, plus specifically targeted therapeutic exercise.

During the growth years through our early 20s, bones automatically command the brain to make extra calcium. Individual diet and health history plays a huge role in meeting the required dose of calcium, even in our youth. Adequate levels of calcium intake will maximize the positive effect of physical activity on bone health during the growth period of children.

The amount of bone tissue in the skeleton, known as bone mass, will keep growing until about age 20. At that point bones have reached their maximum strength and density, which is called peak bone mass. Peak bone mass is influenced by a variety of genetic and environmental factors.

Genetic factors that you are born with, like your gender and race, account for up to 80% of your bone mass make-up, while environmental factors like diet and exercise habits, account for the remaining 20%.

The two key factors that affect our bones as we grow older are the peak bone mass that we've accumulated and the amount of bone loss that has occurred since we achieved our peak bone mass.

Key to the prevention of osteoporosis is to maximize peak bone mass. An important secondary step for prevention is to slow the rate of bone loss as we get older. After the growth years bones require sufficient stimulus from specific exercises targeted to commanding our bodies to demand extra calcium for bone strength. Lack of exercise and inactivity will very likely increase the risk of fracture and simply taking vitamins cannot make up for bad eating habits and lack of exercise.

During my 30s, even though I led an active life and took calcium supplements, I was unaware of two key requirements to keep bones healthy—vitamin D to help the body absorb calcium and the right exercises. I believed that practicing an active lifestyle, like walking to and from work every day, was exercise enough.

In fact, what I needed were specific exercises targeted toward individual bone maintenance and health, which would have strengthened my bones at a time when they were rapidly weakening.

Myth No. 3: Traditional Weight-Bearing Exercises Build Bone Density

Traditional weight-bearing exercises like walking can protect and maintain bone density, but cannot build bone. Activities that build bone are vital to our bone health once we've reached the 40s. Therefore, it is essential to include a variation of three physical activities in your routine:

1. *Weight-bearing* exercises are activities on your feet, with your bones supporting your weight. Examples include brisk walking, dancing, stair-climbing, and low-impact aerobics.

2. *Strength training* includes the use of free weights, weight machines, resistance bands, or water exercises to strengthen the muscles and bones in your arms and spine.

3. *Flexibility* routines increase the mobility of your joints and improve posture. They include regular stretches, Tai Chi, and yoga.

Although each activity alone has some positive impact, all three activities combined in one training routine maximize bone health. Like muscles, bones must be challenged to grow stronger.

If you have osteoporosis or a fracture, consult with your physician and a reputable physiotherapist about the exercise routine best for your body type. During my mid-30's and early 40's I walked about two miles to and from my desk job in the city. I falsely believed that this was a healthy enough routine. Today I've integrated bone and muscle-building exercises that improve my postural alignment and lessen the stress on my spine.

Myth No. 4: Now that I am Older, it's too Late to Have Healthy Bones

As our bodies age, we learn to live with their increasing aches, pains, and maladies. We expect them and accept them with complacency. Often, the thought of exercising the recommended 40 minutes daily is too much to fathom. However, positive health change is possible—if only by taking one baby step at a time. A good way to get started is to make minor changes in small increments: 10 minutes of daily exercise, eating one more vegetable or piece of fruit a day, attending a fitness class, walking to the corner store, or going for a swim. Higher levels of sports activities and household chores along with fewer hours of sitting are associated with a significantly reduced risk for hip fracture in the elderly.

As for nutrition, simply taking the prescribed daily supplement of calcium and vitamin D reduces rates of bone loss in the elderly by 43%. In the frail elderly, activity to improve balance and confidence can help prevent falls. Studies have shown that the elderly who practice Tai Chi have a 47% decrease in falls and 25% of the hip fracture rate of those who do not.

Just like that slight turn in the steering wheel that takes you in a different direction, small changes in your lifestyle can lead to major benefits. The key to successful change is wanting it. The pain I suffered from five spinal fractures made it unbearable to get out of bed in the mornings. Instead of lying there commiserating with myself about the pain, I slowly moved over to the bed's edge and took a breath. Then I rolled one leg over the side of the bed and placed my foot on the floor and took another breath. After several incremental movements I had accomplished my goal.

Today I have the strength and flexibility to get out of bed with little effort or pain.

Myth No. 5: Osteoporosis Is a Natural Part of Aging & Will Not Affect My Lifestyle.

Unlike other diseases, osteoporosis provides no prior physical warnings. There are no aches, pains, or swelling. Instead one day, as for me, a slight wrong movement brings excruciating pain and a lifetime of disability. The timing was poor for me. I'd recently given birth to my first child and was in the throes of early motherhood and at the peak of my career. I am small boned and was aware of my risk for the disease later in life, but never imagined it would strike at such an early age. Continuing in my roles as a wife, mother, daughter, and sister became an insurmountable challenge that I found myself failing to meet. The effects of the disease knew no boundaries and slammed into my lifestyle, bringing it to an immediate halt.

Myth No. 6: My Physician Will Diagnose the Condition Before Any Physical Harm Comes To Me

As many as four out of five people who have osteoporosis are unaware they have the disease and are at serious risk for fracturing a bone. Diagnosis for spinal fracture is a worldwide problem. According to the International Osteoporosis Foundation, only one-third of spinal fractures are diagnosed and treated.

In 2010, Osteoporosis Canada (OC) and the National Osteoporosis Foundation (NOF) released updated guidelines for osteoporosis. The guidelines provide physicians with clear and accurate information to assist them with identifying and assessing patients who are at risk for developing osteoporosis and counseling them on treatment and therapies. OC and the NOF continue to address the challenges of ensuring physicians adopt the guidelines and at-risk patients are aware of the importance of discussing treatment plans with their health care professionals. The latest guidelines for osteoporosis diagnosis and management can be viewed at www.osteoporosis.ca and at www.nof.org

My story is not unusual; women who may be at risk for osteoporosis because of family history, prior medical conditions, or other factors should be tested much earlier in life than is the current practice. Women are usually tested for bone density in their 50's or later—many years after it's too late and bone density is critically impaired. Instead, in my view, they should be tested in their early 40's, making them aware of potential problems and offering treatment and therapy options that could prevent future catastrophic consequences.

Myth No. 7: Young Females Are Safe from Osteoporosis

Premenopausal women who exercise too much or suffer from eating disorders can also develop long-term problems with weak bones when their body weight is so low that normal menstrual periods cease. Excessive athletic training for women over a long period of time for certain sports, like gymnastics or dance, can put them at high risk for osteoporotic fractures, even in their teen years. Teens and older women athletes who train regularly to the point of exhaustion, severely restrict their diet in fear of gaining weight, and workout so strenuously that they no longer menstruate, put their bodies under severe stress. The bone-building process is no longer in balance and the bones begin losing density at a rapid rate. The more bones break down and become weak, the more they become susceptible to fracture.

Myth No. 8: Only Women Get Osteoporosis

One out of eight men will develop osteoporosis from genetics and lifestyle-related causes, or both. Many, like woman, will suffer from a fracture. Men with a strong family history of osteoporosis are more likely to develop the disease, particularly if they smoke and live a sedentary life. By adding exercise to their lifestyle, these men will have a better chance of maintaining bone health. If they stop smoking they can reduce the risk by half. Women are more aware of the disease because twice as many women as men over age 50 suffer from osteoporosis.

Myth No. 9: I Have a Family History of Osteoporosis But I Can Prevent It With Exercise & a Healthy Diet

In Myth No. 2, I discuss how one key growth factor that affects our bones as we age is our peak bone mass. Everyone has a biologically determined peak bone mass with genetic factors like gender and race accounting for roughly 80% of bone mass. A woman, because of her genes, may be destined to have a normal peak bone mass. However, if she has a poor diet that excludes exercise she may only achieve 80% of her potential peak bone mass. In contrast, another woman may be diligent about maintaining her bone health through diet and exercise but, because of genetic factors, have a lower peak bone mass than women the same age. Both women are at risk for osteoporosis. The key to prevention of osteoporosis is to maximize peak bone mass (as it is the reservoir that we will draw upon as aging and other forces affect our skeleton) and slow the rate of bone loss as we get older.

The myths outlined in this chapter are common within the general population and, unfortunately, they also influence many in the health field. Most of us usually visit a doctor with a specific complaint we want addressed. Even if it does occur to us to ask for a bone density test, we may feel too uncomfortable to make the request. So it is no surprise that four out of five people with osteoporosis have no idea that their bones are weakened. Remember— your bones belong to you.

The next two chapters will give you an idea of some of the risk factors associated with osteoporosis, a personal checklist of risk to fill out, the types of tests used to assess bone health, and information to help you get the most out of a medical appointment.

CHAPTER 3

~

THE SILENT DESTROYER: OSTEOPOROSIS RISK FACTORS

One day in 2001 I strolled into a nearby pharmacy and found a nurse offering heel ultrasound bone health tests. I wasn't in a hurry, so why not? The results shocked the nurse conducting the test. She advised me to see my physician, which I did. He requested a bone density test (BMD) and advised me not to be alarmed as heel ultrasound machines are not always accurate. The day of my BMD I was asked by the technologist if there might be any chance that I might be pregnant. I didn't think so, but after a quick discussion we agreed that it might be better to wait until I was absolutely sure that I was not pregnant. Sure enough, I was pregnant! I was unable to have a BMD as the dual rays pass over the abdomen and might put my baby at risk. Instead, they gave me a BMD of the hip (but not the spine) so as to avoid potential harm to my daughter. The BMD results of my hip were good.

Three lessons learned:

- The heel ultrasound can be a first step to assessing your bone health and can help support the need for a BMD

- Bone density can vary in different parts of the body. I did not know that the bone health of my spine could be poor even though the hip was within normal range. We only tested my hip, so the lower bone density in my spine didn't show up

- Trabecular bone, the main component of the vertebrae of the spine, is often affected first.

Step 1: Assess Your Risk for Fracture

Osteoporosis is not necessarily linked to gray hair or retirement. Osteoporosis Canada (OC) recommends that physicians should assess all women and men over age 50 for risk factors for osteoporosis and fracture to identify those at high risk for fractures. In my view, the time for you to assess your bone health is now, regardless of age.

Bone health is a partnership between patient and physician. A little homework before the first visit is a tremendous jumpstart to recovery. An average doctor visit in North America lasts 22 minutes—a brief time to cover such a complex disease.

Before your first visit with a physician to discuss your individual bone care needs and questions, it's important to understand that the health care industry breaks the disease down into two types, *primary osteoporosis* and *secondary osteoporosis*.

Many women have a general understanding of the different causes for osteoporosis. Perhaps there's an elderly relative who appears to be in perfectly good health, whose recent fall has left her with a fractured hip and disabled for months. Or, there could be a friend who is undergoing medical treatment for cancer who is now suffering from severe back pain. In the medical world, the elderly relative who has fallen and fractured a hip is most likely suffering from primary osteoporosis, while the friend who is undergoing treatment for cancer could be suffering from a fracture caused by secondary osteoporosis.

Primary Osteoporosis

Primary osteoporosis is the most common form of the disease, accounting for about 90% of the cases found in women. A number of conditions can cause primary osteoporosis:

- Postmenopausal—the result of a rapid loss of bone due to the decline in estrogen levels during the three to five years preceding menopause (also known as perimenopause); during menopause; and after menopause. Normally though, bone loss occurs at the fastest rate during the first few years after menopause and then begins to level off. Women can lose about 3–5% of their bone mass per year for the first five years after menopause, and about 1% each year thereafter. A decrease in the overall strength of bones gives way to fractures, most often of the wrist and spine.

- Age-associated—a slow decline in bone mass is a normal occurrence in both men and women over age 70, due to the changing balance between the rate of bone breakdown and new bone formation. While a person who has strong and dense bones may not be affected by this gradual bone loss, someone with low bone density could be at risk. Hip fractures are typical for age-related osteoporosis.

- Idiopathic—a term that means the cause is unknown. Idiopathic osteoporosis, which is rare and due to unknown causes, can affect men and women of any age.

Secondary Osteoporosis

Secondary osteoporosis, which accounts for about 10% of cases in women, is traced to one or more underlying conditions, diseases, or medications that affect the bone-building process and disrupt bone formation. As the focus of a health care team is often on the primary disease such as cancer, bone loss and bone fractures are frequently overlooked complications of many diseases and medications. (The questionnaire I prepared in this chapter lists many "secondary" factors that are bad for your bones.) Complete, up-to-date lists of conditions, diseases and medications that contribute to osteoporosis and fractures can be found on these websites: Osteoporosis Canada (www.osteoporosis.ca) and The National Osteoporosis Foundation (www.nof.org).

No matter what your age and your bone situation, improving your bone health is possible. Before you can outsmart osteoporosis and live a future fracture free, you must first gain a better understanding of your bones and body and why you may have developed the disease that has begun to make its mark on your bones. Osteoporosis is a complex condition affecting both bone quality and bone mass, leading to an increased susceptibility to fractures. Although most of your bone strength is genetically determined, many other factors including medical, nutritional, and lifestyle also influence bone.

While the research is contradictory and sometimes confusing, in my view there is sufficient evidence to indicate that the items I have listed in the questionnaire in this chapter can increase the risk of bone loss and fractures. I recommend that you complete this questionnaire, talk to your doctor about your risk for weak bones and fracture, and ask for a bone density test.

Five components of risk-assessment:

1. Hereditary factors (no control).
2. Medical conditions, chronic disease, and some disabilities (no control).
3. Prescribed Medications (may or may not have control).
4. Nutrition and diet (control).
5. Lifestyle factors (control).

A Gallup survey performed by the National Osteoporosis Foundation revealed that 75% of all women aged 45-75 years have never discussed osteoporosis with their physicians.

The following risk assessment can be taken by women at any age.

Osteoporosis Risk Factors Checklist

Explanation of Risk Factors

All of the items listed over the next pages are warning signs or "red flags" that you could be at risk for weak bones and fracture. It is vital to understand how each of these factors can affect your bones. I have seen some of these listed in questionnaires as risk factors (but not all) and they are rarely accompanied by a clear explanation. So, after you finish your risk assessment, I have summarized the research for you. Also, it is important to note that some risk factors are stronger predictors of bone loss than others. Certain factors increase the risk of fracture independent of BMD, the most important being the presence of a prior fragility fracture after age 40 and recent prolonged use of glucocorticoids. (To see the risk factors in 2010 *Clinical Practice Guidelines* go to the OC site www.osteoporosis.ca. or www.nof.org). Check any of the boxes that apply to you and discuss them with your doctor. Each checked box means you have added risk.

Hereditary Factors & Things You Cannot Change

❏ I am a woman

❏ I am 65 or older

❏ I am Caucasian or Hispanic

❏ My hair and skin colour are fairly light

❏ A family member or relative has osteoporosis or has broken a bone as a result of the disease (e.g., your mother, grandmother, sister or aunt fell and broke her hip)

❏ I have broken a bone after the age of 40 without major trauma (e.g., a minor fall versus a car accident)

❏ I have had to be in bed for an extended period of time

❏ I have periodontal disease and experienced tooth loss

❏ I am petite, have a small body frame, and small bones

❏ I am underweight for my height

❏ I weigh less than 60 kilograms (132 pounds)

❏ I have lost more than six cm (about 2.4 inches) in height

❏ I am in menopause or past menopause

❏ I started menopause before age 45

❏ I experienced surgically induced menopause (removal of the uterus and the ovaries)

❏ I have had surgery to remove my ovaries before my periods stopped

❏ I stopped menstruating for prolonged periods of time (more than 3 months at a time—other than because of pregnancy)

Medical Conditions & Chronic Diseases

I have one or more of these medical conditions or diseases:

❏ Cancer

❏ Celiac

❏ Chronic kidney or liver disease

❑ Chronic obstructive pulmonary disease (COPD)

❑ Crohn's or other inflammatory bowel disease

❑ A chronic disease that affects the kidney's, liver, pancreas, lungs, stomach, intestines or hormone levels

❑ Cushing's syndrome

❑ Cystic fibrosis

❑ Depression—major

❑ Diabetes

❑ Eating disorder (anorexia nervosa or bulimia)

❑ Hyperthyroidism

❑ Hyperparathyroidism

❑ Multiple sclerosis

❑ Parkinson

❑ Rheumatoid arthritis

❑ Scoliosis

❑ Vitamin D deficiency

I Take One of These Medications:

❑ Acid suppressing medication including Proton pump inhibitors (PPI) i.e., Nexium and Prevacid and others; Histamine-2 receptor antagonists (H2Ra) e.g., Zantac and Pepcid and others.

❑ Antacids for digestive problems (regular use of those that contain aluminum)

❑ Anti-convulsants, antiepileptic medications (i.e., Dilantin or Depakote)

❑ Anti-depressants (selective seratonin reuptake inhibitors)

❑ Blood thinners (i.e., Coumadin or Fragmin)

❑ Cancer treatments (radiation, chemotherapy)

❑ Contraceptives (Projestin-based i.e., Depro-Provera)

❑ Gonadotropin releasing hormones (GnRH) used for treatment of endometriosis

❑ Steroids (oral glucocorticosteroids i.e., cortisone or prednisone for asthma or arthritis)

❑ Thyroid medicine

You're nearly done!

Things you Can Change

Nutritional Factors

❑ I have had less than two servings of dairy products in my daily diet over the years

❑ I have very few calcium-rich foods in my daily diet

❑ I have had little vitamin D in my daily diet over the years

❑ I diet frequently

❑ I dieted sporadically in my teenage years

❑ I am lactose intolerant

❑ I drink more than four cups of beverages that contain caffeine each day—coffee, tea or cola

❑ I drink soft drinks daily

❑ I consume foods high in protein and sodium every day

Lifestyle Factors

❑ I am not active or able to be active

❑ I walk less than 20 minutes per day

❑ I sit most of the day

❑ I don't do bone-building exercises (i.e., brisk walking, aerobics, weights or resistance bands)

❏ I am or was a smoker

❏ I have more than seven alcoholic beverages per week

❏ I have trained as an athlete and have experienced absence of menstruation from over-exercising

❏ I have poor vision

❏ I have poor balance

❏ I sometimes fall

Hereditary Factors & Things You Cannot Change

Gender

Your risk of developing osteoporosis is greater if you are a woman. In general, women have smaller, thinner and less dense bones than men, putting them at greater risk of developing the disease. Also, owing to the decline in estrogen during and after menopause, women lose bone more rapidly than men. It may surprise you to know that osteoporosis is a significant health problem for men as well, although it often develops about 10 years later than in women.

Age

The risk of osteoporosis grows as you grow older. Your bones naturally become weaker and less dense as you age. However, osteoporosis is a decrease in bone mass greater than expected for a person's sex, age, and race. Risk rises at about age 50 and sharply increases at age 65.

Racial Origin/Hereditary Factors

Family history of osteoporosis and fracture plays a role in your bone health. For example, if your mother broke her hip, you are at higher risk of breaking your own hip.

Caucasian and Asian women are more likely to develop osteoporosis since their bone density is often lower than that of African-American women, Hispanic women, or women of

Mediterranean or Aboriginal decent. Women with fair skin, freckles, or red or blond hair are at higher risk for the disease. The reasons why women from one ethnic background are more at risk than others are not yet clear. While hereditary paleness puts you somewhat more at risk, it is important to know that 80% of those affected by osteoporosis are women from all ethnic backgrounds.

Health & Bones

My mother broke her hip

Knowing your parents health history is important. A parental history of fracture, especially hip fracture, is a risk factor for you for osteoporosis.

I have broken a bone while an adult

Osteoporosis is often a "silent" disease until it causes a fracture. A broken bone in the wrist, hip or spine from minor trauma is often the first symptom. If you break a bone after the age of 40, talk to your doctor immediately about measuring the density of your bones and develop a plan to improve your bone health. Remember that the consequence of fracture is an increased risk of a subsequent fracture.

I have had to be in bed for an extended period of time

Bed rest is bad for the bones. Like muscle, bone is living tissue that responds to physical activity by becoming stronger. Women who are on prolonged bed rest due to surgery, serious illness, or complications of pregnancy or immobilized due to stroke, fracture, spinal cord injury, or other chronic conditions often experience a significant bone loss. When inactive, our bone turnover accelerates. Our skeleton responds to immobilization by a rapid and sustained increase in bone resorption (bone being dissolved) and a more subtle decrease in bone formation (bone-building) due to increased osteoblast function. Stress and the forces we put on our bones through physical activity stimulate bone cells, which improves bone strength and inhibits bone loss with age.

I have periodontal disease and experienced tooth loss

Women don't often associate osteoporosis with their "pearly whites" and a trip to the dentist but they should. Osteoporosis can increase tooth loss and periodontal disease and periodontal disease in women may indicate the presence of osteoporosis. If the jaw bones that anchor your teeth start losing density you are at more than 80% greater risk of having gum disease, which is the major cause of tooth loss in women over 35. And bone around the roots of the teeth tends to erode quickly when calcium is depleted from the body. Individuals with osteoporosis suffer more tooth loss than people without the disease.

Body size, height, and weight

Women with small bones weighing under 132 pounds are at greater risk for osteoporosis and fracture for they have less bone mass to draw upon as they age. Also at risk for fracture from a fall are slender women with a low body weight for their height as they tend to have less bone mass and less muscle padding than medium-frame or larger women. Yoyo dieting can also wreak havoc on your bones. When you lose weight you also lose fat, muscle, and bone density. Fat and muscle may come back, but bone could be gone forever.

Loss of height

Height loss may be the first sign of osteoporosis. Bad bones can lead to broken vertebrae in the spine. Because broken vertebrae in the spine don't always cause pain, height loss may be the first sign of bone loss. If you have lost more than 6 cm (2.4 inches), the loss being the difference between the tallest height you recall being and your current measured height, you may have a spinal fracture.

Hormonal factors

Menopause is mean to your bones. The leading cause for osteoporosis in women is the drop in estrogen levels that occurs during menopause. Menopause, whether natural or surgically induced, leads to the body producing less estrogen (and the ovaries stop producing estrogen) which leads to rapid bone loss. The hormone estrogen helps suppress osteoclast (the cells that breakdown bone) activities.

Lack of estrogen enhances the ability of osteoclasts to absorb bone and limits the absorption of calcium needed for osteoblasts to build bone. When the bone-removing osteoclasts do their job better than the bone-building osteoblasts, the net result is bone loss.

In the absence of estrogen, a woman absorbs calcium less well and excretes it more vigorously.

Women who have premature menopause (before the age of 45) tend to get weaker bones faster than women who enter menopause later in life.

Women with amenorrhoea—the absence of a period for more than three months (apart from pregnancy or breastfeeding)—experience significant loss of estrogen, which leads to premature and rapid bone loss.

Conditions & Medications

While the research is contradictory and sometimes confusing, there is sufficient evidence to indicate that the following conditions and medications can increase the risk of osteoporosis and fractures. Anyone with one or more of these conditions or who uses one or more of these medications should talk to a physician immediately. Request a bone density test, confirm the correct doses of calcium and vitamin D, and inquire about the proper exercise routine.

Use of the medications listed in the checklist below can increase your risk of fracture. Do NOT stop taking your medication—you are on it for a reason, rather than a possible risk. Instead, consult your regular doctor, whose knowledge of your health and prescription history makes her or him best equipped to assess your bone health and determine if you are at risk for fracture. The information presented here is intended to complement, not substitute, the expertise and judgment of your physician, pharmacist, or health care professional.

Medical Conditions & Chronic Diseases

Cancer

Cancer survivors have an elevated risk of osteoporosis and fractures. Cancer itself can be bad for the bone-building process. Powerful chemotherapy drugs and estrogen-blocking hormone treatments are highly effective in treating cancer but they can be harmful to the bones.

Women with breast cancer, the most common female cancer in North America, may be particularly at risk if they are treated with an aromatase inhibitor (AI). Since most breast cancers are estrogen-dependent, these drugs are used to suppress estrogen. These drugs cause bone loss by reducing the amount of estrogen in the body. While lowering levels of estrogen is beneficial in treating cancer, it is harmful to bone health since estrogen helps bones stay strong.

Celiac

Osteoporosis can be the first sign of untreated celiac disease—an intestinal disorder in which the body can't tolerate gluten. Gluten is a protein found in wheat, rye, barley, farina and bulgur. When people with celiac disease eat foods that contain gluten, their immune systems respond by attacking and damaging the lining of the small intestine. As the small intestine is responsible for absorbing nutrients, when the lining is damaged the nutrients in food such as calcium and vitamin D, which are essential for healthy bones, cannot be properly absorbed into the blood stream for the body to use.

Chronic kidney or liver disease

Kidneys keep minerals in the body in balance, including the ones that help keep bones healthy. Weak and brittle bones and fractures are prevalent among women with chronic kidney disease. Bone loss occurs in kidney failure patients because of hormonal deficiencies, lack of weight bearing exercise, improper diet, alcohol abuse, insufficient vitamin D, and the effect of glucocorticoid medications to treat the diseases.

If calcium levels in your blood become too low due to kidney failure, a hormone called parathyroid hormone (PTH) will begin removing calcium from your bones to get calcium blood levels back to normal. As calcium is stripped from the bones, they can become weak, more like a piece of chalk than a sturdy bone.

Extra phosphorus is another bone stripper. It is normally removed from the body by healthy kidneys, but when your kidneys don't work, phosphorus builds up in your blood. Healthy kidneys create activated vitamin D, called calcitriol. When kidneys fail, they stop converting inactive vitamin D to calcitriol. The result is your body is unable to absorb calcium from food, so it "borrows" the calcium it needs from the greatest calcium storage depot — your bones.

Nutrients, hormones, drugs, and poisons are not processed effectively in women with chronic liver disease (CLD). In addition, protein production and other substances produced by the liver are inhibited. CLD is shown to increase the prevalence of osteoporosis in postmenopausal women, particularly in the lumbar spine. Increased bone resorption seems to be the main reason and the osteoblasts can't keep up and fill the bone cavities. Calcium malabsorption may occur in patients with chronic liver disease due to malnutrition, vitamin D deficiency, and the use of glucocorticoid treatment.

Chronic Obstructive Pulmonary Disease (COPD)
Patients with COPD often become aware of their osteoporosis only at their first fracture due to the lack of awareness of the connection between COPD and osteoporosis. COPD is a group of diseases of the lungs that make it hard to breathe. Cigarette smoking is the most common cause of COPD. Emphysema and chronic bronchitis are the two main conditions that make up COPD. Medications used to treat people with COPD as a well as smoking, vitamin D deficiency, and decreased activity as the disease progresses all play a role in bone loss in COPD patients.

Crohn's disease and other inflammatory bowel diseases
The incidence of fracture among persons with inflammatory bowel disease (IBD) is greater than that in the general population. As an example, up to 60% of people with Crohn's disease have low bone density. People with an IBD, which causes inflammation in the digestive tract, often have difficulty absorbing calcium and vitamin D—two key bone builders. In addition, the glucocorticoid medications often used to treat these diseases can lead to bone loss.

Cushing's Syndrome

Cushing's syndrome is a disorder that develops when the body makes too much of the so-called "stress" hormone cortisol. However, the most common cause is from taking cortisone-like drugs called glucocorticoids (such as prednisone for arthritis) for more than three months. Too much cortisol is bad for the bones as it hinders calcium absorption, leading to weak bones and potential fracture.

Cystic fibrosis

Cysric fibrosis (CF) is a hereditary disease that affects the mucus glands of the lungs and the digestive system. In the lungs, CF causes severe breathing problems. In the digestive tract, CF makes it extremely difficult to absorb nutrients including calcium and vitamin D. Also, inadequate physical activity and the use of glucocorticosteroids to treat CF can contribute to thinning of bones and increased risk for fracture.

Depression

Bad moods can lead to bad bones. Although the link between the brain and the bones is a new area of study, researchers have found that there is a connection. Ongoing depression can lead our bodies to make chemicals which are detrimental to the bone-building process. Depression and some of the drugs to treat it can lead to bone loss. Other behaviours linked to depression can also be detrimental to bones including: increased smoking and alcohol consumption, reduced physical activity, poor nutrition, and reduced exposure to sunlight (low vitamin D) due to more time spent in doors. Depressed women are less likely to exercise, eat a well-balanced diet, and care for their general health and well being.

Diabetes

Type 1 diabetes, once known as juvenile diabetes or insulin-dependent diabetes, is a lifelong condition in which the pancreas produces little or no insulin. Insulin is a hormone needed to help sugar (glucose) move from the blood into the body's cells, where it can be used for energy or stored for later use.

Women with type 1 diabetes have lower bone mass, increased risk for fracture and longer healing periods after fracture than women without the disease. There is a definite link, but researchers are still not sure why. Postmenopausal women with type 1 diabetes have a higher rate of hip fracture than those without the disease.

Type 2 diabetes, once known as adult-onset or noninsulin-dependent diabetes is a similar—although much more common—condition in which the body becomes resistant to the effects of insulin or the body produces some, but not enough, insulin to maintain a normal blood sugar level.

Because Type 2 diabetes is associated with obesity, risk of fracture is higher due to a sedentary lifestyle and poor coordination and balance. Vision problems and nerve damage associated with the disease can also increase the risk for falls and broken bones.

Eating disorders (anorexia nervosa or bulimia nervosa)

Anorexia and other eating disorders assault bone health. People with anorexia have an intense fear of being fat, an extreme fear of weight gain, and a distorted view of their body size. People with anorexia restrict their food intake by dieting, fasting, or excessive exercise. Bulimia is similar to anorexia. With bulimia, a person binge eats (eats a lot of food) and then tries to compensate in extreme ways, such as forced vomiting or excessive exercise, to prevent weight gain. Although anorexia and bulimia are very similar, people with anorexia are usually very thin and underweight but those with bulimia may be a normal weight or even overweight.

Eating disorders impair bone health because of two major factors. Most women with eating disorders have irregular or no menstrual periods which causes a drop in estrogen which leads to premature bone loss. Secondly, lack of proper nutrition is common, with poor intake of bone builders including calcium and vitamin D.

Since eating disorders commonly begin during the teenage years, this poses a special risk as it can mean the failure to reach peak bones mass which puts a person at greater risk for fracture throughout their life.

Hyperthyroidism/hyperparathyroidism

Hyperthyroidism is a condition in which an overactive thyroid gland is producing an excessive amount of thyroid hormones that circulate in the blood. Overactivity of the thyroid gland, whether it is caused by the gland itself or too much thyroid replacement medication, can cause bone loss.

When you are hyperthyroid, osteoclasts (the cells that remove old bone) get over-stimulated. They begin to remove old bone faster than it can be replaced by the osteoblasts, which are not affected by the excess thyroid hormone. You wind up with too much bone removed and subsequent bone loss. (*The Thyroid Source book for Women* online by M. Sara Rosenthal)

The four powerful parathyroid glands located behind the thyroid gland regulate calcium levels in the body so the nervous and muscular systems can function properly. We store many kilograms of calcium in our bones and it is readily available to the rest of the body at the request of the parathyroid glands. If one of the glands develops a benign tumour it can become overactive (hyperparathyroidism) and too much PTH hormone is secreted. This causes our bones to release calcium constantly into the blood stream resulting in a loss of bone density and hardness (it is the calcium that makes bones hard).

Although the thyroid gland and the parathyroid gland are close together and have an impact on our bones they do not affect each other's levels of activity.

Multiple Sclerosis

Multiple Sclerosis (MS), which is three times as likely to occur in women than in men, is a condition in which the immune system attacks the central protective myelin covering of the central nervous, system which can affect vision, hearing, memory, balance and mobility. People with MS suffer more fractures compared to healthy women. Lack of physical activity, poor balance, and the corticosteroid medication sometimes used to treat MS can lead to poor bone health.

Parkinson's disease

Parkinson's is a nerve disorder that causes tremors, difficulty moving, muscle rigidity and balance problems. People with Parkinson's are at increased risk for fracture because of decreased mobility and higher tendency to fall.

Rheumatoid arthritis

It is important to distinguish between two very common forms of arthritis—rheumatoid arthritis and osteoarthritis. They are two very different medical conditions with little in common, but the similarity of their names causes great confusion. These conditions develop differently, have different symptoms and are diagnosed and treated differently.

Rheumatoid arthritis (RA) is an inflammatory condition where enzymes released in the body destroy the lining of the joints (an area in the body where two bones meet) in the body causing pain, stiffness and swelling. Bone health is affected by both the disease and the drugs to treat the disease. Both can provoke an increase in osteoclast activity which can lead to bone loss. In addition, if the disease leads to inactivity, further bone loss can result.

Osteoarthritis is a painful, degenerative joint disease that develops when cartilage (the smooth covering over the bones in your joints), starts to break down usually as a result of aging, trauma, or increased wear and tear.

While it is possible to have both osteoporosis and arthritis studies show that people with osteoarthritis are less likely to develop osteoporosis. People with rheumatoid arthritis may be more likely to develop osteoporosis, especially as a secondary condition from drugs used in treatment.

Scoliosis

Scoliosis and kyphosis refer to abnormal curvatures of the spine. With scoliosis the spine bends unnaturally to one side or the other causing compression of one side of the body. Kyphosis, is an exaggerated forward bend of the upper spine and looks like poor posture or a rounded or humped back. Women with osteoporosis are more vulnerable to scoliosis and other deformities of the spine and women with scoliosis are more vulnerable to osteoporosis. Scoliosis can be caused by genetic conditions, leg length inequality, degeneration of the discs and joints between the vertebral bodies, a spinal fracture or a combination of these problems. Kyphosis can be the result of degenerative diseases, such as arthritis of the spine, compression fractures of the vertebrae caused by osteoporosis, or trauma to the spine.

Vitamin D deficiency

Vitamin D deficiency is an unrecognized worldwide epidemic. Many people know they need calcium for their bones but many women are unaware of how vital vitamin D is to our skeleton. Vitamin D, which is obtained from sun exposure, our diet, or supplements is essential to absorb calcium from food in the intestines and helps to form and maintain strong bones as it stimulates bone remodeling. Inadequate production and intake of vitamin D—or deficiencies caused by liver or kidney disorders or other diseases—leads to muscle weakness, increased osteoclast activity, and accelerated bone turnover leading to thin and brittle bones. Vitamin D is responsible for the recruitment of osteoclasts. Not only that; vitamin D also plays an important part in the mineralization of bone matrix. Due to these two important roles that vitamin D plays, a lack of it can result in the whole bone renewal process being compromised. Research shows there is a link between high vitamin D intake and high bone density.

Medications

Acid suppressing medication

Using certain medications for more than one year to treat gastroesophageal reflux and peptic ulcer diseases commonly known as heartburn and indigestion puts your bones at risk for fracture. Proton pump inhibitors (PPI) i.e., Nexium and Prevacid and others; Histamine-2 receptor antagonists (H2Ra) e.g., Zantac and Pepcid and others suppress gastric acid which is required to absorb calcium. Poor calcium absorption can speed up bone mineral loss and lead to fractures.

Antacids

Regular use of over the counter antacids that contain aluminum (e.g., Maalox and Gaviscon), used to treat mild digestive problems, are bad for your bones. Aluminum has a toxic affect on calcium and interferes with the body's ability to absorb calcium.

Anticonvulsants, antiepileptic medications

Drugs used to control epilepsy, a condition with repeated seizures, put women at risk for weak bones. Anti-epileptic drugs, also called anti-convulsants such as Dilantin or Depakote, work by slowing down impulses in the brain that cause seizures. Unfortunately they can also impair absorption of calcium.

Anti-depressants (selective seratonin reuptake inhibitors)

People aged 50 and over who regularly took anti-depressants called selective serotonin reuptake inhibitors (SSRIs) such as Prozac, Paxil, or Zoloft, had double the rate of fractures as those not using these medications. SSRIs, which are prescribed to treat depression, anxiety or post traumatic stress disorder, affect the bone-building process so the longer women are on SSRIs, the weaker their bones become.

Blood thinners

A class of medications called anticoagulants that are commonly referred to as blood thinners serve to prevent and treat blood clots in the veins, arteries, and lungs. These drugs hamper vitamin K in the body as it helps make blood clots. Drugs such as Coumadin or Fragmin are used to thin the blood to decrease the amount of clotting that occurs. However, studies have shown that vitamin K is needed, along with calcium and vitamin D, for making and keeping our bones strong.

Cancer treatments (radiation, chemotherapy)

Cancer survivors who have received therapy are at elevated risk for fracture. Treatments for cancer, known as aromatase inhibitors (AIs), such as Arimidex, Aromasin, and Femara suppress the production of estrogen in the body, leading to bone loss. Canadian and American breast cancer guidelines now recommend that women with risk factors for osteoporosis who are taking AIs undergo a bone mineral density test.

Contraceptives (Projestin-based i.e., Depo-Provera)

Depo-Provera increases osteoporosis risk according to a Health Canada release in July 2005. Depo-Provera, commonly prescribed for contraception and for treating endometriosis, contains a powerful variant of the hormone progesterone which is known to cause bone loss in women of all ages and reduce peak bone mass in adolescents when they are in the critical stage of bone growth. The longer the drug is used the greater the risk for weak bones and fractures.

Gonadotropin releasing hormones (GnRH) & Nafarelin

Gonadotropin releasing hormones (GnRH) act the same ways as the body's own hormones while Nafarelin is a man-made protein that has the same effect as a GnRh. They are used for treatment of endometriosis, a condition where tissues which should only be located inside the uterus find their way elsewhere in the body. The most common symptom of endometriosis is pelvic pain. GnRH interferes with estrogen production—and we know that bone density diminishes as estrogen levels drop.

GnRH effectively makes you "menopausal" for the time that you use the treatment. Endometriosis is fed by estrogen and without the estrogen stimulation, endometriosis shrinks down and becomes inactive. Examples of GnRH agonists include: Zoladex, Synarel, Suprecur and Prostap. The aim of these medications is to reduce or stop the estrogen being produced in a woman's body, so that it does not continue to feed the endometriosis growths.

Steroid hormones

Glucocorticoids (distinct from the anabolic steroids used by body builders) are widely used to treat a number of medical disorders such as severe allergies, skin problems, asthma, immune system diseases (i.e., rheumatoid arthritis or muscular dystrophy), and to prevent and treat rejection of transplanted organs. They mimic hormones secreted by the adrenal cortex and are often referred to as corticosteroids.

Excess corticosteroids decrease calcium absorption, decrease bone formation, increase bone resorption, and increase fracture risk of the hip and spine.

Thyroid medicine

Excess thyroid hormone medicine accelerates the breakdown of bone (stimulates bone destroying cells) which is detrimental to the bone-building process. It is a risk factor for bone fracture for peri- and postmenopausal women.

Things You Can Change

Nutritional Factors

Calcium

Calcium is critical every day over your lifetime for your bones, teeth and total body health. 99% of your body's calcium is stored in your bones. Children and teenagers need adequate calcium in their diets every day so they can maximize the calcium storage in their bones. In later years, adequate dietary calcium helps minimize calcium loss from the bones. Studies show that over half of North Americans do not get the recommended calcium from their diets. The average person loses 400 to 500 mg of calcium per day through normal bodily processes such as waste, shedding of hair, fingernails, perspiration, and skin. If a woman's diet does not include enough calcium to replace what is used, the body will take calcium away from the bones, which weakens them and makes them more likely to fracture.

Your body borrows calcium daily from your bones for your blood to use. But it also redeposits calcium regularly from the food you eat, so new bone is continually being formed. As we get older, it gets harder for our bodies to absorb calcium—just when we tend to be eating less and in general taking in less calcium in our diets.

Vitamin D

Evolution designed us to get most of our vitamin D from sun exposure, but nature didn't take into account our indoor lives and northern winters. This is why 50% of North Americans don't get enough vitamin D. So the vitamin D we take in from such foods as eggs and milk is very important.

Vitamin D is crucial for calcium absorption. Your body's need for both minerals increases as you get older. Even if you do consume a lot of dairy, you may want to talk to your doctor about taking a vitamin D supplement, just to be sure your calcium absorption levels are at their peak.

Dieting

Studies show that too few calories can disrupt the reproductive system and impair bone formation in teens and college-age females. If a young woman's menstrual cycle stops, it is considered a warning sign of bone loss.

Maintaining proper weight is important to overall health, but so is good nutrition. If a young girl is avoiding all milk and dairy products and severely restricting her food intake, she is probably not getting enough calcium. She needs a more balanced diet that includes low-fat milk products and other calcium-rich foods. Calcium supplements may also be helpful to ensure that she gets enough of this essential nutrient.

Lactose intolerance

One of the primary risk factors for developing osteoporosis is not getting enough calcium in your diet. Because dairy products are a major source of calcium, you might assume that people with lactose intolerance who avoid dairy products could be at increased risk for osteoporosis. However, research exploring the role of lactose intolerance in calcium intake and bone health has produced conflicting results. Some studies have found that people with lactose intolerance are at higher risk for osteoporosis, but other studies have not. Regardless, people with lactose intolerance should follow the same basic strategies to build and maintain healthy bones and should pay extra attention to getting enough calcium.

Caffeine

More than 400 milligrams of caffeine a day from a source high in caffeine (such as coffee, soda pop, energy drinks, hot chocolate, over the counter pain medications, chocolate bars, and even ice cream) may cause us to excrete extra calcium in our urine. Caffeine is a diuretic and it increases the amount of calcium we excrete in our urine for several hours after we drink it. This is cause for concern for those with osteopenia or osteoporosis. We should not be doing things that will reduce the amount of calcium we absorb. Research also shows that caffeine may interfere with the absorption of vitamin D which is necessary for the body's absorption and use of calcium.

Soft drinks

Studies suggest that drinking sodas (diet or regular) can limit the calcium you'll have available. Most sodas contain phosphoric acid and calcium, magnesium, and phosphorus must be maintained in the proper balance for bone health. When too much phosphorus is in the blood, calcium is leached from the bones, causing osteoporosis. One survey found that women who drank carbonated drinks had more than twice as many broken bones as those who didn't drink soda.

Lower intakes of calcium and magnesium have been accompanied by a large increase in the consumption of non-diet sodas. Twenty years ago, the average teen drank as much milk as soda. Today, teens average twice as much soda as milk.

Adolescence is a critical time for bone development and any factors that have a detrimental affect on the bone-building process at this age can have long-term consequences. The chance one will have osteoporosis in later years is related to the amount and density of bone at the completion of growth.

Protein

Eating too much protein or too little protein is bad for the bones. Too much protein, compared to the amount of calcium consumed, increases calcium loss in the urine which can lead to bone loss. Taking in more animal protein than you need causes your body to create organic acids that acidify the bloodstream. The kidneys neutralize the acidity by pushing large amounts of calcium into the urine. Calcium may also be pulled from the bones to neutralize the acid created to digest large amounts of protein.

The average person needs 60-75 grams of protein a day (one gram per kilogram of body weight.) There are no exact numbers, but too much protein is probably defined as more than three or four times this amount.

On the other hand, one study showed that women who didn't meet their needs for protein had severe bone loss. So both eating too much protein and too little protein cause osteoporosis.

Ensuring adequate calcium intake (through a sufficient intake of dairy foods, or calcium supplements) is crucial for bone health when large amounts of protein are being consumed.

(An excellent resource on nutrition and bone loss can be found at the website of the US Surgeon General: *Other Nutrients and Bone Health At A Glance.* http://www.niams.nih.gov/Health_Info/Bone/ Bone_Health/Nutrition/other_nutrients.asp.)

Sodium

Pass on the salt. Sodium affects the balance of calcium in our bodies by increasing the amount we excrete in urine and perspiration. The loss of calcium can be significant. The more salt you eat, the more calcium leaves your body.

The National Institutes of Health, a component of US department of Health and Human Services, recommends restricting daily sodium intake to less than 2,400 mg (equal to about 1 teaspoon of salt). Most people innocently exceed this limit through foods that they do not know contain salt, including cereals, convenience and pre-packaged foods, pizza, subs, hamburgers, hotdogs, soup, canned vegetables, and pasta.

Lifestyle Factors

Physical Activity

Use it or lose it. If you don't stay active and exercise you lose bone mass and muscle strength. The best types of exercise for bone health are weight-bearing and strength training as they help keep bones strong and prevent calcium loss.

Weight-bearing exercise includes brisk walking, tennis, running, soccer, dancing, and aerobics.

Strength training includes free weights, machine weights, resistance machines, resistance or elastic bands and can stimulate bone-building.

Another benefit of staying active is that regular exercise helps improve balance and coordination and can reduce risk of falls and fracture.

Smoking

The chemicals in cigarettes are toxic to the bones. Smoking reduces calcium absorption and slows down the activity of bone-building cells, which increases your risk of broken bones. Women who smoke have lower estrogen levels and earlier menopause. We know estrogen deficiency accelerates bone remodeling, so that bone is broken down faster than it is formed. Women who smoke, particularly after menopause, have a significantly greater chance of spine and hip fractures than those who don't smoke.

Alcohol Consumption

Drinking more than seven alcoholic beverages per week can increase your bone loss. Alcohol in large amounts is directly toxic to osteoblasts, thus reducing bone formation, and may also directly affect bone mineral density by impairing liver function and interfering with the absorption and use of calcium and vitamin D. It is a double hit—the bones become weaker and we become physically clumsier under the influence, making a fall and resulting fracture more likely.

Falls

Falls lead to fractures and can be fatal. The statistics are alarming. Over 90% of hip fractures are caused by falling, most often by falling sideways onto the hip. About 76% of all hip fractures occur in women. About one out of five hip fracture patients dies within a year of the injury. Up to 25% adults who lived at home before the hip fracture had to stay in a nursing home for at least a year after their injury.

The afternoon I received the call from my physician to tell me that I had five fractures in my spine I was stunned. Although I went through a battery of tests, no one really could determine why my bones had gone bad by the early age of 42. I have since gone over the preceding risk factors and can see what could have wreaked havoc on my bones:

1. Bad bones run in my family. I was genetically predisposed. My maternal grandmother and aunt each had a hip fracture. My mother was diagnosed with osteoporosis in her 70's. All developed the dowager's hump—the infamous sign of fractures in the spine before bone density testing existed.

2. During my pregnancy it was discovered that I was at risk for blood clots and was required to give myself daily injections of a blood thinner for six months.

3. Bed rest, the bone robber, was also required for eight weeks during my pregnancy due to placenta previa (the placenta covered the cervix and caused bleeding which was risky for both me and the baby).

4. Hindsight is 20/20. I am certain that I never truly attained a solid peak bone mass and therefore went into the pregnancy with less than robust bones.

5. I am fair skinned, small boned, slender, and weigh 125 pounds.

6. I have a curvature in my spine due to the left leg being shorter than the right leg (since birth).

7. In my 20s and 30's I did include some calcium and minimal vitamin D in my diet but nothing close to the daily requirements that were required to maintain good bone health. At that time there was no general awareness of the need for vitamin D to help absorb calcium.

8. Although I walked to work and was active, I did not focus on bone-building exercises such as weights or resistance bands. In my 30s, to climb the ladder of success, I worked many hours sitting at a desk, computer, or in meetings.

CHAPTER 4

~

A TRIP TO THE DOCTOR: WHAT TO ASK & WHAT TESTS TO EXPECT

I have spent a lot of time with doctors and other health care professionals since I found out I have osteoporosis. I saw my family doctor 3-5 times before a trip to the ER revealed my spinal fractures. Then I had visits with various specialists, stays in hospital, physiotherapy, massage therapy, etc. Suddenly, medical appointments took over my life. At first, I had no idea what to expect or what to ask. I just wanted the pain to stop. I soon realized that I needed to be prepared at each visit—otherwise I might have to wait months to ask a vital question.

Unfortunately, I found that most of the books and literature are written from the perspective of the physician and for the physician, which made it difficult because I wanted information from a patient's perspective. The good news is, after months of combing through materials from many, many resources and working with physicians, advocates of osteoporosis, and other patients who've suffered from the disease, I gathered enough information to have done your homework for you!

The week I sat down to write this chapter, I had just returned from an appointment with one of my doctors. Having had more than 50 medically-related appointments over an 18-month period following my fractures, I've put in a lot of hours at the doctor's office. With all the experience, trial and error has taught me hundreds of strategies and tips for maximizing your bone health appointments. These have been narrowed down into the most important and itemized in the following pages.

Remember, if you suspect you are at risk for or have been diagnosed with osteoporosis, the cause of the disease may not be the result of one factor, but the cumulative effect of a number of factors from the risk assessment tests that apply to you. Once diagnosed with the disease, it is imperative to review every possible contributing factor, and then develop a comprehensive plan with a health care team to manage and improve your bone health. For example, your physician may concentrate on medication options, but not have time to discuss specific exercises to improve your bone health. It's up to you to ask questions and ask for help in the areas specific to your plan, like diet and exercise.

We all know how time crunched doctors are. To make the most of the minutes you do get with your doctor it is imperative to do your bone health homework and prepare for your appointments.

There are three critical steps to making the most out of your bone health check ups:

1.   Assess your risk for fracture (Chapter 3 checklist).

2.   Prepare for an appointment with your doctor.

3.   Know what to expect.

Prepare for an Appointment with Your Physician

The goal of assessing your risk for fracture (hopefully, you have completed the questionnaire in Chapter 3 by now) is to manage your bone health and prevent a fracture. Once you fracture your chances of future fractures are extremely high. Your target goal is to minimize or slow the rate of bone loss as you age—the sooner the better.

The main obstacle to early diagnosis of the disease is the lack of symptoms and pain until a fracture has occurred and the disease is well advanced. Occasionally, even fractures do not cause any pain.

There have been many scientific advances in osteoporosis research in recent years, but current clinical practice does not always reflect application of the knowledge. Many high-risk patients continue to be undiagnosed and untreated.

Therefore, it is in your best interest to do the homework and come to the appointment prepared with specific questions and concerns.

Osteoporosis affects the shape and architecture of your bones.

In some cases, it is fairly easy for a physician to detect osteoporosis, usually when it's severely progressed. This is the biggest single issue with osteoporosis. Simply put, physicians treat symptoms and more often than not, there are no symptoms until the disease has advanced to the point of brittle, fragile bones. If the disease is to be diagnosed before it reaches this point, there needs to be a better understanding of its predictors, which we learn by taking the risk assessment test in Chapter 3.

Figure 4.1: Pictures of healthy and osteoporotic bone

Normal bone   *Osteoporotic bone*

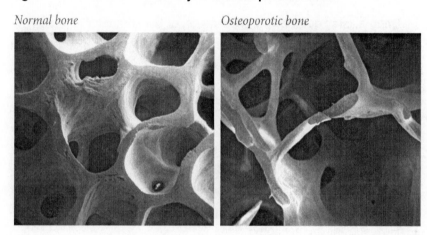

Use the information from your risk assessment test to prepare for a visit with the physician. Now you have the knowledge base to work with the physician to target your specific bone health plan, which should be a partnership between you and your health care team.

With the average physician visit being so short, it's essential that the patient be prepared and armed with the knowledge to work with the physician to create a health care plan that is beneficial to future bone health. Therefore, it is important to do your homework in order to get the most out of your medical visits and play an active role in improving your bone health.

After taking the risk assessment test, whether you are at high risk or no risk at all, your bone health should be, at the least, addressed with your physician as early as your next visit.

Medical Visit Preparation Check List

Complete the Risk Assessments in Chapter 3.

❑ Know your family's medical history.

❑ Bring a list of symptoms and their frequency, duration, and intensity.

❑ Bring a list of medications, doses, and length of time you have been taking them.

❑ Estimate the amount of calcium and vitamin D you get daily through diet and supplements.

❑ List any allergies to food or medications

❑ Prepare to honestly answer questions about your lifestyle, including weekly exercise, alcohol, and caffeine intake.

❑ Bring a list of questions and concerns, or both, in order of priority.

❑ Be prepared to take notes and take a moment to summarize and repeat everything you were told by the doctor.

❑ Bring a friend or family member to help take notes and provide support.

Ask:

❑ For a copy of the results of your bone mineral density test and what it means in terms of your risk of fracture.

❑ For results of other tests and what they mean e.g., blood test for vitamin D level.

❑ How you will be monitored.

❑ Who you can contact after the appointment if you have questions.

❑ When you should schedule your next appointment.

❑ If you should see a specialist like a rheumatologist or endocrinologist.

❑ If physiotherapy is right for you and for the name of a reputable physiotherapist if you are experiencing physical pain.

❑ For exercise recommendations or a reliable contact for one if you have limitations.

❑ How much calcium and vitamin D to take.

❑ What different types of medications are available and those the physician would recommend for your bone health

❑ If there are any tests or medication(s), or both, you will need and which are covered by your province or state health insurance plan.

Know What to Expect: Bone Health Tests

Now that you've completed the five-part assessment in Chapter 3, and prepared for your appointment with the doctor, it is to your advantage to understand how you will be examined and what tests are available to determine your bone health.

Undergoing a bone check-up requires patience on the patient's part because the doctor will need to perform one or more of several tests to diagnose your bone health. The physician's challenge is to target tests specific to your needs and collect and interpret the results. Each test result is analyzed and the information compiled for your file, like putting together pieces of a puzzle.

The physician's goal is to assess your bone strength. Bone strength encompasses both bone quality and bone density. Bone mineral density (BMD) refers to the amount of mineral in a given area of bone and is assessed relatively easily. However, there is no precise definition of bone quality, nor is there an established mechanism available to the public for measuring it. When health professionals use the term bone quality, they refer to bone architecture, mineralization, rate of turnover and accumulation of damage.

Bone Mineral Density Measurements

Bone mineral density (BMD) measurements are the gold standard tool for diagnosing osteoporosis. Although it is still a very important piece of the puzzle in the bone health check up, recent research shows that BMD alone is insufficient to predict the risk of breaking a bone. There are some women with BMD results just below normal who have experienced a fracture. As a result, doctors are to look at all other risk factors for low bone mass and fractures listed in clinical guidelines for osteoporosis to help assess bone health.

According to the National Osteoporosis Foundation (NOF), fracture risk is now looked at in an entirely new way. The NOF *Clinician's Guide* released in 2010 provides evidence-based recommendations to help healthcare providers better identify people at high risk for developing osteoporosis and fractures and assuring that those at high risk are recommended for treatment to lower the risk. The *Clinician's Guide* applies the algorithm on absolute fracture risk by the World Health Organization (WHO). This algorithm estimates the likelihood of a person to break a bone due to low bone mass or osteoporosis over a period of 10 years. In addition, absolute fracture risk calculations help to resolve much of the uncertainty about management for people with low bone mass (osteopenia), the precursor to osteoporosis. The NOF has estimated that more than 10 million Americans have osteoporosis and an additional 33 million have low bone density of the hip. Recognizing the difficulty in measuring bone mass and bone quality accurately and determining how to best treat and manage patients with low bone mass, the WHO developed the Fracture Risk Assessment Tool (Frax) to assess individual 10-year fracture risk. Also, the NOF has expanded its guidelines beyond Caucasian postmenopausal women to include African-American, Asian, Latina, and other postmenopausal women.

According to Osteoporosis Canada (OC), since the publication of their guidelines in 2002 there has been a paradigm shift in the prevention and treatment of osteoporosis and fractures. The focus is now on preventing fragility fractures and their negative consequences, rather than treating low bone mineral density which is viewed as only one of several risk factors for fracture. Current data suggest that many patients with fractures do not undergo appropriate assessment or treatment. To address this care gap for high-risk patients, the 2010 guidelines concentrate on the assessment and management of women and men over age 50 who are at risk of fragility fractures and the integration of new tools for assessing 10-year risk of fracture into overall management.

Visits to the doctor are essential for your bone health. Examinations and tests can be worrisome when you don't know what to expect. To ease your apprehension I have summarized several tests physicians carry out to determine and manage your bone health (Table 4.1). Physicians often cover the following: a detailed medical history, physical examination, biochemical tests, BMD, and a 10-year risk of fracture probability. Now let's take a look at these and other possible bone health tests in more detail.

Table 4.1: Bone Health Tests

Test Type	Test Reason
Questionnaire	Fracture risk Primary or secondary osteoporosis
Physical exam Height Rib-pelvis distance Weight	Risk for bone loss Possible fracture
Biochemical tests (Blood and urine samples)	Determine baseline levels of substances Quality of bone: bone turnover Response to treatment
Bone Mineral Density (BMD)	Density of bone
X-rays	Fractures
FRAX or CAROC	10-year risk of a fracture
Other tests: Bone scan, quantitative computed tomography (CT), magnetic resonance imaging (MRI), bone biopsy and quantitative ultrasound (QUS)	May be requested to further investigate bone loss, fractures or other bone conditions

Test Type—Questionnaire

To determine fracture risks, the doctor will usually begin with a medical history. He or she may ask you to fill out a questionnaire and inquire about your family history of osteoporosis or fracture, and past and present health care concerns with any of the risk factors you have already determined, based on your self-assessment. This is an ideal opportunity to address the results of your risk-assessment, any concerns you may have regarding primary or secondary causes of bone loss and a treatment plan that would optimize your bone health.

Test Type—Physical Exam

After questions and routine tests, the doctor will conduct a physical exam, recording your skeletal build as small, medium, or large, and your height and weight. Height is a good baseline because patients with compression fractures in the spine will lose their height. And low body weight (less than 60 kg or 132 lbs) or major weight loss is an important risk factor for osteoporosis and increased risk of fracture.

He or she may also examine posture and measure leg length. Poor posture, curvature of the spine, leg length differences, an awkward gait, and severe back pain are signals of the possibility of osteoporosis and fracture(s).

The importance of height measurement cannot be overemphasized. According to OC, measurement of height should be routine physician procedures for adults, especially for those over 50. Spinal fractures affect more than 50% of all women and one sure way to detect them is height loss.

Physicians should always record your height as a matter of routine office visits, and as you age note any height loss from previous visits and historical height loss. If you have lost more than 2 cm (over any timeframe up to three years) there is a possibility that you have had a spinal fracture. Historical height loss is the difference between the tallest height that you recall being and your current measured height. Historical height loss greater than 6 cm (2.4 inches) suggests that vertebral fractures are present. Therefore, it's essential when managing your bone health, to inquire about height loss during routine physician visits.

Physicians also can perform a rib-pelvis distance (RPD) test to assess spinal fractures. My vertebral fractures are in my lower back (lumbar spine) and are not as noticeable as multiple fractures might be in the upper back. My physician, however, can confirm the presence of fractures by measuring the vertical distance between the bottom of the ribs and the top of the pelvis. An RPD of less than two fingerbreadths strongly suggests the existence of a vertebral fracture, most likely within the lumbar spine.

Test Type—Biochemical

Blood and urine tests are helpful to the physician assessing your bone health and risk for fracture. Bone density changes so slowly that BMD tests usually don't show results for a year or more. Doctors can monitor your response to treatment more quickly using blood or urine tests.

Substances that are detected in the urine or blood may serve as a sign of a disease or other abnormality. More often blood samples are taken (and sometimes urine samples) to determine a baseline level for all biochemical markers, and then repeated later to monitor response to treatment over time. Biochemical markers are any hormone, enzyme, antibody, or other substance that is detected in the urine, blood, or other body fluids or tissues that may serve as a sign of a disease or other abnormality.

Throughout the skeleton, thousands of microscopic sites, called remodeling units, are busy dissolving old bone and replacing it with new bone. The process is essential to repair and replaces old, and damaged bone that has microscopic cracks. In resorption, osteoclasts, which we'll call excavators for purposes of understanding them better, are called such because they go to work to resorb old, damaged bone tissue.

Figure 4.2: Bone Remodeling Process

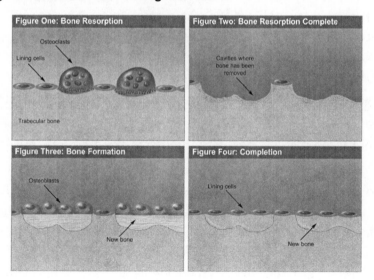

It takes an estimated two to four weeks for the osteoclasts to do their job, and a then a few months for the osteoblasts to complete their work. If the bone remodeling rate changes, there is a so-called "uncoupling" of the osteoblasts and osteoclasts, which cripples them from doing their job. This is when the bones begin to break down and in correlation, risk for fracture increases.

One example is in menopause, where studies have shown that the rate of bone remodeling can double at menopause because of the decline in estrogen. When bone turnover increases, the new bone is not formed fast enough to replace the old bone that has been removed.

During bone turnover, substances are released into the blood stream. These are biochemical or "bone" markers. More often blood and sometimes urine samples provide physicians with key information about your bone turnover rate and determine how rapidly osteoclasts are breaking down bone, and how effectively osteoblasts are at restoring new bone. For example, high levels of bone turnover markers are associated with high rates of bone loss in postmenopausal women.

Urine is tested for calcium content and for components associated with bone resorption. If the calcium content in your urine is too low, it may mean you are absorbing calcium from your diet less effectively. If your calcium content is too high, it can be a sign that the calcium is being robbed more rapidly from your skeleton. Abnormally high levels of certain substances in a urine sample can be a warning sign that you may be losing bone density too rapidly.

As the main role of vitamin D is to help regulate the absorption of calcium it too may be measured through a blood sample to ensure you have adequate levels of vitamin D.

To date, bone markers have been very useful for research to determine the onset of drug action but they are not yet routinely used for diagnosis and management of osteoporosis. However, doctors may choose to review bone markers to help diagnose osteoporosis and identify "fast bone losers" and patients at high risk of fracture.

Test Type—Bone Mineral Density (BMD)

A bone mineral density, or BMD, may be one of the most important tests you take when determining the health of your bones. Because of this, I want to spend some time on:

What is a BMD?

Why a BMD is needed?

Who should get a BMD?

Making sense of the BMD report.

What Is a BMD?

A bone mineral density test measures how many grams of calcium and other bone minerals, which are collectively known as bone mineral content, are packed into a segment of bone. The higher your mineral content, the denser the bone. And the denser your bones, the stronger they are and the less likely to break.

There are a number of devices on the market that are used to measure bone mineral density. They include dual photon X-ray absorptiometry (DXA), quantitative computerized tomography (QCT) and ultrasonometry (QUS). DXA is the most widely accepted and widely used technology and considered the gold standard today. Bone Mineral Density tests are quick, painless, noninvasive, and safe.

Why Is a BMD Needed?

A low bone density score is an important determinant of fracture. As with any test in our health care system, health practitioners have to weigh the cost and availability of equipment to perform the BMD tests. So in lieu of mass screening, health care guidelines target men and women who are at high risk for developing osteoporosis and who are at risk for fracture. So the first question to be asked for who to test for a BMD is who is at risk for fracture? This question is somewhat like the one that asks, "Which comes first, the chicken or the egg?" because the purpose of a BMD is to determine if you are at risk for fracture. So prior to asking for a BMD, it is essential that the patient is at risk for bone loss and fracture.

Who Should Get a BMD?

If I could set a national health care policy for all women at the age of 40 to get a BMD test to determine a baseline and assess their bone health, I would. However, this is not economically feasible in many countries because of the limited number of bone density machines and staff available to perform the test and meet with patients to discuss the results.

The National Osteoporosis Foundation and Osteoporosis Canada recommend that all post menopausal women and men age 50 and older should be evaluated clinically for osteoporosis risk in order to determine the need for BMD testing. And that patients, who in consultation with their physicians discover that they are at high risk of developing osteoporosis, have a BMD in order to plan for a proper health care strategy. The conditions for a BMD from the OC 2010 *Clinical Practice Guidelines for the Diagnosis and Management of Osteoporosis in Canada* are listed in 4.2.

Table 4.2: Conditions for a BMD Test

Adults ≥ 50 years	Adults < 50

• All women and men age ≥ 65 years
 	
• Menopausal women, and men aged 50-64 years with clinical risk factors for fracture:
 	
  - Fragility fracture after age 40
 	
  - Prolonged glucocorticoid use
 	
  - Other high-risk medication use (see www.osteoporosis.ca)
 	
  - Parental hip fracture
 	
  - Vertebral fracture or osteopenia identified on X-ray
 	
  - Current smoking
 	
  - High alcohol intake
 	
  - Low body weight (< 60 kg) or major weight loss (>10% of weight at age 25 years)
 	
  - Rheumatoid arthritis
 	
  - Other disorders strongly associated with osteoporosis
	• Fragility fracture
	
	• Prolonged use of glucocorticoids
	
	• Use of other high-risk medications (see www.osteoporosis.ca)
	
	• Hypogonadism or premature-menopause (age < 45 years)
	
	• Malabsorption syndrome
	
	• Primary hyperparathyroidism
	
	• Other disorders strongly associated with rapid bone loss and/or fracture

Table adapted from http://www.osteoporosis.ca/multimedia/pdf/Quick_Reference_Guide_October_2010.pdf

At present there is no one true measure of overall bone strength. Bone mineral density is frequently used to measure bone health and accounts for approximately 80% of bone strength.

How Is the BMD Report Read?

Many people I know have had a BMD and are familiar with the term but few have understood what it is and how to interpret the results.

A bone density test measures how much mineral is found within the bone and it is reported in grams per square metre (g/cm2). Once bone density is measured, it is compared to that of an average young adult (T-score) and to the average of an individual the same age and gender (Z-score). The average young adult reading compares your density to the optimal peak bone density of a healthy young adult of the same sex.

The age-matched reading compares your bone mineral density to what is expected of someone of your age and, sex. The information from a bone mineral density test enables the doctor to identify where you stand in relation to others your age and to young adults, which is presumed to be your maximum bone density. Scores significantly lower than "young normal" indicate you have osteoporosis and are at risk for bone fractures.

The results also assist the doctor in the best way to manage your bone health, as BMD is used to assess response to treatment.

The difference between your BMD and that of a healthy young adult is referred to as a standard deviation (SD). The World Health Organization (WHO) has recommended that BMD measurements be reported using T-scores to define normal bone mass, low bone mass (or osteopenia), and osteoporosis.

As most fractures occur in people who have osteopenia, not those with osteoporosis, early identification of low bone mass is crucial.

Table 4.3: Making Sense of BMD Reports
(sources: the International Osteoporosis Foundation and Osteoporosis Canada)

Classification	Statistical Meaning	What it really means
Normal	T-score of-1 or better Bone density is no more than 1 standard deviation below the young adult normal value	Your bone density is average or better than that of young adult woman and within a healthy range. 85% of young adult woman are in this range
Osteopenia (low bone density)	T-score between-1 and-2.5 Bone density is 1 standard deviation to 2.5 standard deviations below the young adult normal value	Warning sign. Your bone density is below the normal range but not low enough to be considered osteoporosis. The lowest 1-14% of healthy young adult women have bone density this low
Osteoporosis	T-score of-2.5 or poorer Bone density is more than 2.5 standard deviations below the young adult normal value	You have osteoporosis. Your bone density is significantly lower than the normal healthy range. It is lower than 99% of healthy young adult women
Severe osteoporosis	T-score of-2.5 or poorer and a fragility fracture Bone density is more than 2.5 standard deviations below the young adult normal value and there have been one or more fragility fractures	You have osteoporosis and you have at least one fragility fracture

As BMD decreases fracture risk increases. For each standard deviation decrease in BMD fracture risk almost doubles.

Table 4.4: Making Sense of BMD Reports, Your Z-score

(Source for Table 4.4: *Strong Women Strong Bones 2000*)

Z-score	Statistical Meaning	What it really means
Higher than-1	Your bone density is within 1 standard deviation of the average for women your age, or better	Your bone density is within or above the normal range for a woman your age
Between-1 and-2.5	Your bone density is between 1 and 2.5 standard deviations lower than the average for women your age. Warning sign. Your bone density is lower than average for your age	Warning sign. Your bone density is lower than average for your age
Less than-2.5	Your bone density is lower than 2.5 standard deviations than the average for women your age	Your bone density is significantly lower than the average- lower than 99% of women your age

The frequency of BMD tests will depend on your risk for fracture. The coverage for BMD tests varies across provinces and states so be sure to check with your physician and health insurance coverage prior to the test. However, even if it is not covered by your health insurance policy, in my view it is worth investing in the test.

Test Type—X-Rays

X-rays are not helpful in the early diagnosis of osteoporosis. Although they can detect fractures, they cannot detect osteoporosis until the bone loss is well-advanced. When evaluating women for osteoporosis, a doctor will suggest an X-ray if a fracture in the spine or other area such as the wrist is suspected. X-rays are better at assessing one type of bone (cortical) over another (trabecular). We will get into the different types of bones in Chapter 5. For purposes of explaining why X-rays are not helpful in an early diagnosis of osteoporosis, understand that osteoporosis predominantly affects trabecular bone and X-rays don't reveal changes caused by osteoporosis until cortical bone is affected. Cortical bone is not affected until osteoporosis is reaching an advanced stage, where 25-40% of bone loss has occurred.

I can't stress strongly enough how important it is to remember that there are spinal fractures that do not cause enough pain to warn of their presence. Other factors such as height loss might lead your doctor to request an X-ray as it can be helpful to detect fractures in the vertebrae in the spine and serve as a baseline for future X-rays. Also, the radiologist may be able to tell whether the spinal fracture is old or recent.

According to Osteoporosis Canada (OC), spinal fractures are the most common type of osteoporotic fracture and they are underdiagnosed and inadequately followed up. OC recommends that radiologists report all spinal fractures seen on chest X-rays, regardless of the initial purpose of the examination, and, where appropriate, make recommendations for further evaluation.

Test Type —FRAX or CAROC-10–Year Fracture Risk

There has been wide media coverage about a new fracture risk assessment tool called FRAX, developed by the World Health Organization (WHO). FRAX is a simple web-tool that takes key information and risk factors and plugs them into a formula to predict a 10-year probability of major osteoporotic fracture for both women and men worldwide. The model for each country has been created using data from the country's population. It is a practical tool that has been created using data from populations in various countries. FRAX is a system for determining absolute fracture risk. Different FRAX tools are needed for each country since fracture rates are very different, even between the United States and Canada.

FRAX was designed to assist in the better targeting of women and men in need of intervention, and in the improved allocation of limited healthcare resources toward patients most likely to benefit from treatment.

There is one statistic which I found incredibly shocking. First, as many as 50% or more fragility fractures (*Reversing Osteopenia* 2004) in postmenopausal women actually happen when bone mass T scores are in the osteopenia range, not the osteoporosis range. This means that women with osteopenia may need to consider treatment options. In other words, an incredible number of fractures occur before osteoporosis is even present. This is why it is so important not just to look at BMD to assess your risk of fracture and whether to be treated for osteoporosis. Health professionals don't always agree about when to start medications for osteopenia. Some believe that prevention must start early and others are more conservative and believe that more evidence is required that early treatment actually prevents fractures before prescribing treatment. My opinion is this, you want to do everything you can to prevent that first fracture for once you have a spinal fracture your chances of another spinal fracture in the first year are five-fold and you have a higher risk of a hip fracture. If you have osteopenia, read Chapter 3 to see if you have any other risk factors and determine your 10 year probability of a fracture with your doctor and discuss the best course of action.

Fragility fracture defined

According to Osteoporosis Canada, it is a fracture occurring spontaneously or following minor trauma such as a fall from standing height or less.

A bone is considered osteoporotic if it has lost density to the point that it is unable to withstand the traumas of normal activities or if the bone has fractured already from minor trauma. For example, a healthy person may have a minor trip and during the fall, by instinct, use their hands to brace the fall. A person with healthy bones may experience bruising or pain while a person with osteoporosis could suffer one or two fractured wrists.

The NOF's *Clinician's Guide* applies the algorithm on absolute fracture risk (FRAX). Absolute fracture risk calculations help to resolve many of the questions about management for people with low bone mass, also called osteopenia. These are individuals with a T-score between-1.0 and-2.5 on their bone mineral density (BMD) test.

According to the NOF, physicians clearly knew in the past to treat people with osteoporosis, that was not the case for people with osteopenia. Now these people and their doctors have information from absolute fracture risk methodology to determine when it is medically appropriate to treat, and when it is not, based on the likelihood of breaking a bone. It is important to note that the WHO algorithm is for untreated patients to help decide when to treat, and does not apply to patients already taking an osteoporosis medication. You can go to the FRAX website (www.sheffield.ac.uk/FRAX/), choose the country you are from, and complete the questionnaire entering your factors (for example, having broken a bone, being a smoker or on a steroid medication) as well as bone mineral density (BMD) at the hip. The FRAX tool then calculates your 10-year risk of hip fracture and your 10-year risk of a major osteoporotic fracture (i.e., spine, forearm, or hip).

Currently, two closely related tools are available in Canada for estimating the 10-year risk of a major osteoporotic fracture: the updated tool of the Canadian Association of Radiologists and Osteoporosis Canada (CAROC; see www.osteoporosis.ca) and FRAX as explained above but specific for Canada. At the time this book was released, software for the Canadian version of FRAX was not yet widely available on BMD machines; therefore, for purposes of reporting BMD, the 2010 version of the CAROC tool was the only system that could be applied across Canada.

Other Tests

In most cases, all of the above pieces of the puzzle can be put together and your doctor can adequately assess your bone health. In some cases, the results may spur your physician to order further tests to explore your bone health. These other techniques that are less widely used for the diagnosis and management of osteoporosis and fractures include: bone scans, quantitative computerized tomography (CT), magnetic resonance imaging (MRI), bone biopsy, and quantitative ultrasound (QUS).

Bone Scan

Although the term is often interchanged, a bone scan is not the same as a BMD. A bone scan is a nuclear scanning test to find abnormalities in bone and monitor conditions that affect bones. It is primarily used to help diagnose a number of conditions relating to bones, including: cancer of the bone or cancers that have spread to the bone; unexplained bone pain such as ongoing lower back pain; broken bones such as a hip fracture or a stress fracture not clearly seen on X-ray, and detecting damage to bones due to infection or illness.

For a bone scan, a small amount of a radioactive tracer substance is injected into a vein in the arm. The tracer then travels through the bloodstream and into the bones. "Hot spots" may indicate problems such as arthritis, a more recent fracture, or an infection. A bone scan can often detect a problem anywhere from days to months earlier than a regular X-ray. It can be helpful when it is unclear whether a fracture in the spine is recent or fairly old.

Quantitative Computerized Tomography (QCT Scan)

The only technique available to patients that is three-dimensional, meaning it can be used to measure 100% isolated trabecular bone. All other techniques, such as DXA produce a two-dimensional image and cannot measure pure trabecular bone. DXA measures a mixture of both trabecular bone and the overlying compact bone. The CT scan can give an image of a slice through one or more vertebrae.

Although more accurate than DXA, QCT is mainly used for research and for special cases due to its cost, limited access, and the high dose of radiation required. The radiation for a CT scan of the entire body is equivalent to a thousand X-rays!

Magnetic Resonance Imaging (MRI)

Magnetic Resonance Imaging, better known as MRI, is a method of looking inside the body and producing detailed pictures using magnets and waves, instead of radiation. It can be used to distinguish between recent and old fractures of the vertebrae and stress fractures of the hip.

Overall, the differentiation of damaged bone from normal healthy bone is often better with MRI than with other imaging techniques such as X-ray, CT and ultrasound. The combination of radiowaves and the magnetic field can produce detailed images of the spine and bones, and unlike plain X-rays, an MRI will picture soft tissue such as joint ligaments, muscles, and their tendons.

MRI can check for problems of the bones and joints, such as arthritis, cartilage problems, torn ligaments or tendons, or infection. MRI can also show if a bone is broken if an X-ray cannot. MRI can check the discs and nerves of the spine for other conditions as well.

In many cases, MRI gives different information about structures in the body than can be seen with an X-ray, ultrasound, or computed tomography (CT) scan. MRI may show problems that cannot be seen with other imaging methods.

Bone Biopsy

A bone biopsy is a procedure in which a small sample of bone is taken from the body and looked at under a microscope for bone disorders. A bone biopsy is often done on bone areas that show problems on an X-ray. It confirms the diagnosis of a bone disorder (such as cancer) or checks bone problems that were found by another test, such as an X-ray, CT scan, bone scan, or MRI scan, and find the cause of ongoing bone pain.

The major reason to have a bone biopsy is to rule out other bone diseases. It can, however, be painful, invasive, and expensive. Since many of the other tests, such as BMD and bone markers, can detect osteoporosis without invading the body, bone biopsies play a limited role and are seldom used.

Quantitative Ultrasound (QUS)

Women who are at risk for broken bones do not always have access to the gold standard DXA to test their bones. In fact, many women who should have a BMD test are not getting it. In accordance with the National Report Card released by Osteoporosis Canada in 2009, lack of access and availability of equipment keep people from getting tested, and this is likely to get worse as the population at risk for osteoporosis grows.

As an emerging alternative to DXA, there is a growing interest in the use of quantitative ultrasound (QUS) for the assessment of fracture risk. Whether or not combining QUS and DXA improve fracture prediction is still unclear and needs further research. There is growing evidence to support the use of QUS in osteoporosis and there are now over 8000 ultrasound scans used worldwide.

The test is inexpensive, accessible, fast, painless and because the scan uses ultrasound waves, it does not expose patients or staff to radiation. The equipment is compact and easily trans-portable, therefore ideal to provide a service to the community via pharmacies. By combining the results of a heel ultrasound with known risk factors for osteoporotic fractures, doctors are able to assess which women face a greater risk of fracture. It can be effective at identifying high-risk patients who should receive further testing.

QUS is an option for people who don't have access to the gold standard BMD test in rural and remote areas; elderly women who are unable to lie down on the table for the BMD; and women who have degenerative changes in the spine which can falsely elevate the results of a BMD. The heel is used because we are measuring the trabecular bone—the honeycomb-like part of the bone. This bone deteriorates first in osteoporosis. It is found in largely in the wrist, spine, heel and the hip joint. The heel has mainly trabecular bone, and is therefore an easy site to measure.

In my view, any equipment that can help a woman assess her risk before she breaks a bone is a good thing! QUS can be used as a first step along with a review of risk factors for bone loss to determine if you need a BMD. Doctors can use the results, along with information about family history, diet, age, stage of menopause, and other risk factors to determine the need for further investigation and management.

An ultrasound exam of the heel combined with an assessment of specific risk factors for bone loss and falling can help predict fracture risk due to osteoporosis.

QUS, although more accessible, requires more research and does have limitations. There is no standardized ultrasound test and different medical centers use different machines. Different machines give different readings due to differences in calibration and analysis software used. Unfortunately QUS can't check the bone density in the spine and hip. A test done on your heel may predict risk of fracture in your spine and hip. But because bone density tends to vary from one location to the other, measurements taken at the spine or hip by DXA are considered more accurate assessments of risk for osteoporosis and fracture because these are the bones most likely to break.

Prevention is the best medicine! You are the one with the most to lose if your bones are bad. Advocate for yourself with your healthcare providers.

But let's be realistic—if you are reading this book there is a good chance that you already are diagnosed with osteopenia or osteoporosis. And perhaps, like me, you have suffered a fracture and want information and tips to help you heal and to prevent future fracture. In which case, keep reading.

Chapter 5

~

Spinal Fractures & Osteoporosis

When I heard the alarming news that I had five spinal fractures in my lower back as a result of osteoporosis, I had no idea of the impact it would have on me in the short and long-term. I found it extremely challenging to get the information I needed to understand how my body had been affected by the fractures and what my steps to recovery should be. My orthopedic surgeon, physician, endocrinologist, rheumatologist, physiotherapist, and other health care practitioners had parts of the puzzle but it took a great deal of effort to put all the pieces together to make decisions that were best for me and my body.

I can't stress enough the need to manage life after fracture. Why? Because, whether painful or not, once you fracture, your chance of another fracture is incredibly high. One fractured vertebra puts stress on the spine and can weaken the entire structure. So it is essential to prevent the cascade of fractures and the consequences they may bring. In addition, the fracture itself may not be that harmful to your body but the complications after the fracture may be devastating and have long-term affects.

In writing these chapters I walk a delicate balance between fear and hope. I share some scary statistics to reinforce why it is necessary to take steps to prevent future fractures—even if you have not experienced any symptoms after a fracture. To balance this I have shared some very positive and uplifting information about how to prevent future fractures, maintain or regain independence, and maintain quality of life. Chapters 6 to 19 address the possible physical and emotional effects that come with spinal fractures and more importantly provide a guide map for your road to recovery from one of the most prominent and debilitating consequences of osteoporosis—spinal fractures.

We cannot reverse the damage caused by osteoporosis but we can learn to live well with the disease. We can do things to prevent future fractures and enhance our quality of life. The body has an extraordinary capacity to mend itself. From personal experience, I know that there is a light at the end of the tunnel. But I also know that it can be a lonely, painful time. Sometimes we see no end in sight. At times I felt hopeless, but I somehow managed to keep moving forward towards the vision of the life that I wanted. I gained power and control over my disease.

When my vertebrae fractured I was only 42—younger than most people who get this kind of injury—but my age didn't protect me from the pain and suffering. I needed help. There was plenty of medical information, but very few resources offered practical solutions to the daily challenges of living with spinal fractures caused by osteoporosis. Chapters 6 to 19 of *Unbreakable* are devoted to sharing information and experiences that you can use to recover from fractures and to manage this disease.

I have focused on steps to begin the journey of recovery that are nonsurgical and that take place after diagnosis of a spinal fracture by a health care professional such as a physician or specialist. A spinal fracture is not something you want to self-diagnose! Most people who have vertebral fractures do not have surgery, particularly elderly people, because of the risks associated with both surgery and hospitalization. Although it is a rare option, I have addressed surgical options in Chapter 14 that you may wish to explore further.

Common Osteoporosis Fractures

For many men and women, the first sign of osteoporosis is a fracture—a break in a bone. Worldwide, one in three women and one in five men over 50 will have a fracture caused by osteoporosis in their lifetime (according to the International Osteoporosis Foundation). These broken bones can turn an active life into one of pain, disability and dependence.

Some bones are more vulnerable or are at higher risk for fracture than others because of where they are located in the body or because of the ratio of trabecular to cortical bone.

Almost 80% of your skeleton consists of cortical bone. Cortical bone, the harder protective outer shell (cortex means "tree bark" in Latin) is remarkably thin—in areas such as the femur it can be as thin as two millimetres (.08 of an inch). It is predominant in the long bones of our arms and legs and contributes to the skeleton's strength.

Trabecular bone, the spongy and more porous bone, makes up the other 20% and is made up of thin lattice like struts and is lost twice as fast in osteoporosis compared with the dense cortical bone. Trabecular bone makes up most of the ribs, spine, small bones of the wrist and pelvis. The most common fractures linked to osteoporosis are those of the spine, wrist and hip—the areas where there are significant amounts of trabecular bone. The spine and hip are critical to our balance and mobility, so it is essential that we protect them if we want to enjoy an active life.

Osteoporosis is responsible for more than 1.5 million bone fractures each year in the United States:

- 700,000 vertebral (spinal) fractures
- 300,000 hip fractures
- 250,000 wrist fractures
- 300,000 fractures of other bones

- National Institute of Arthritis and Musculoskeletal and Skin Diseases (US)

Because my personal experience is with spinal fractures and not a wrist or hip fracture, the following chapters address spinal fractures, the possible impact of this type of fracture, and a road map to recovery.

CHAPTER 6

~

THE DIVINE SPINE

T he spine is our body's central structure and tower of strength. Keeping it healthy is vital to our mobility. Unfortunately, we rarely think of our spine and its significance to our daily life functions until it is too late and the damage is irreversible. I know because it happened to me when I suffered spinal fractures simply bending over to lift my newborn daughter from her crib. This was the exact moment when the life that I had known for 42 years came to an abrupt halt. A long, painful, and often frustrating journey to recovery was about to begin. If only I could turn back the clock and know in my 30's what I know now about the spine's dichotomous strength and delicacy.

Healing from my spinal fractures took nine long months that required my husband's help with the simplest daily activities like showering, dressing, and walking from one room to another. Simply bending over the sink to brush my teeth or pulling on a pair of socks were daily challenges that brought me to tears. I dreaded errands outside the house—negotiating any kind of step, getting in and out of a car, and the many trips to and from medical appointments.

We were forced to hire a nanny to care for our infant daughter during the day, as my husband was not available to help during that time. But there was still the tremendous responsibility of caring for her in the evenings. The dependence on a nanny would bring me to an emotional low when, after several months, I noticed a special bond developing between my precious newborn and her caregiver—an intimacy that is usually only shared between a mother and her child. On reflection, I realize that my desire to regain my special bond with my daughter was a huge motivator to get better, and to do so as quickly as humanly possible.

An Information Superhighway

Understanding the spine's intricacies is a critical first step in the prevention of spinal fracture. Where fracture has already occurred, as in my case, it is vital to managing and coping with the crippling side effects and pain.

The human body is built in an amazingly orderly fashion and the spine is no exception. At birth we have more than 300 bones and by adulthood many of them have fused. A mature adult body contains more than 600 muscles and 200 bones. Every one of them is charged with the single role of helping our body's movements.

The spinal cord is a direct extension of the central nervous system from the brain. Made up of a large bundle of nerves, the spinal cord serves as an information superhighway relaying messages between the brain and the body. The spinal cord is enclosed and protected by the bones of the spinal column. The spinal column is approximately 46 cm (18 inches) long and made up of 24 individual bones called vertebrae, which are supported by muscles and ligaments.

- Each vertebra has a hole in the center and is shaped in such a way that when stacked on top of each other like building blocks, they protect the spinal cord and all its nerves. Between each vertebra are shock-absorbing discs that help absorb pressure, prevent bones from rubbing against one another, and give the spine its flexibility. In addition to discs, special joints between each of the vertebral bodies, called facet joints, connect each vertebra to the next. These connecting joints allow individual bones of the spine to move and rotate in tandem

- Ligaments that allow the spine to bend, twist, and carry body weight with the perfect balance of strength and flexibility join the entire spinal column

- Muscles that closely surround the spine bones are important for maintaining posture and assisting the spine during normal activities such as walking, bending, and lifting.

A closer look at a healthy spine and its structure makes it easier to understand how spinal fractures affect the body. As infants we are born with a fairly straight spine. As we grow older and learn to walk our spines develop an "S" shape. The spine's curves work like a coiled spring, allowing the spine to be incredibly strong and highly flexible. Although the lower back holds most of the body's weight, each of the three regions of the spine relies upon the other's strength to function properly. These regions, called cervical, thoracic, and lumbar, are slightly different in composition and shape.

- The cervical spine or neck gradually curves inward at the neck and is made up of seven vertebrae that support the head's weight and allow it to turn from side to side

- The thoracic spine or upper back gradually curves outward in the middle of the spine and is made up of 12 vertebrae. These structures protect the chest organs and have little motion because they are firmly attached to the ribs and breastbone

- The lumbar spine or lower back gradually curves and is made up of five vertebrae in women and six in men. These vertebrae are the largest in the spine because they bear the majority of the body's weight.

Figure 6.1: The Spine

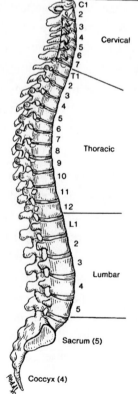

C1
2
3
4   Cervical
5
6
7
T1
2
3
4
5
6
7
8   Thoracic
9
10
11
12
L1
2
3   Lumbar
4
5
Sacrum (5)
Coccyx (4)

Each vertebra is like a well-tuned machine part. If healthy, they support the body and allow load bearing, movement, and bending. However, with just one fractured vertebra the spine's strength is altered. Several fractures will (in most cases) create painful symptoms and permanently alter the shape and strength of the spine.

Fractured Spine. Fractured Life.

Treating spinal fractures is vastly different from treating other broken or fractured bones because of the complexities and central positioning of the spine inside the body. With a broken limb, a cast can be applied directly, immobilizing and protecting it from further injury and giving it time to heal. In some cases of spinal fracture a brace can provide minor protection, but a cast is never an option. Therefore, it is impossible to isolate the spine from irritating activities and daily movements like sitting, walking, or turning over in bed. Spinal fractures present daily physical challenges that were once taken for granted. They can transform an energetic, highly independent person into a spiritless, inactive one who is dependent on others to perform the simplest of normal activities.

The most common fracture associated with osteoporosis is a spinal or vertebral fracture, where one vertebra of the spine is broken. This fracture is so common that one occurs every 12 minutes in Canada. Because vertebrae are made up of softer trabecular bone tissue, they are particularly vulnerable to osteoporosis. For someone who suffers from severe osteoporosis, a fracture can occur from a simple sneeze or an abrupt twisting motion. It can happen from the pull of gravity over time. In my case, a slight movement to lift my baby daughter from her crib fractured my spine in five places. A healthy spine withstands these movements and is only affected by major trauma like a car accident or falling from a ladder.

Spinal fractures range in size and severity from an easily missed hairline crack to a complete collapse of the vertebra. Collapsed spinal fractures are called compression fractures and vary in degree from mild wedges to complete compressions, which occur when the bones of the spine become broken due to trauma. As vertebrae become thin they are prone to collapse from relatively minor forces or breakage in circumstances where extreme pressure is exerted against them. This can result in loss of height and force the spine to fall forward, causing the torso to bend slightly downward at the shoulders, creating a physical appearance oftentimes referred to as "Dowager's Hump."

Figure 6.2 Fractures of the Spine

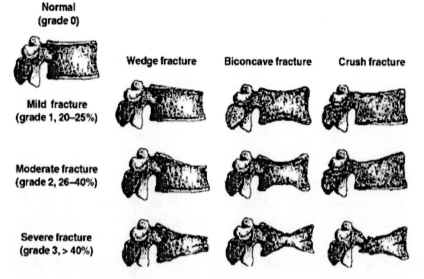

In more severe cases of multiple compression fractures the loss of height can be significant. It causes the rib cage to press down on the pelvis reducing space in the abdomen. My five compression fractures caused heartburn, my stomach to protrude, and enlarged my waistline enough to make it impossible to properly fit into my clothes. I constantly struggled to squeeze into pants and skirts. Extreme cases can also lead to impaired lung function and, with compressed abdominal organs, a reduced appetite that leads to unhealthy weight loss.

Symptoms or Symptomless

About one-third of patients who have vertebral fractures won't experience any symptoms and go undiagnosed. Just because they don't feel the pain that usually accompanies a fracture doesn't mean that they are any less vulnerable to them. A lack of painful symptoms does not eliminate the risk of future fracture and its effect on quality of life. In fact, lack of pain makes matters worse by leaving the patient unaware of any need for treatment or caution. Immediate symptoms of a spinal fracture to watch for include:

- A pop or snap felt or heard at the time of injury

- Difficulty and pain that increases when standing, walking, bending or twisting
- Swelling and bruising in the spinal area
- Limited movement in the spinal area
- Numbness, tingling, or weakness in the arms or legs
- Sudden, severe back pain
- Back pain that increases when pressure is applied to the area.

Confusing Back Pain

Fractures that alter the natural curves in the spine put pressure on the back creating pain ranging from mild to debilitating. Unfortunately nothing can be done to restore the vertebra to a normal state. If the vertebra collapses gradually rather than suddenly due to an activity, the pain is usually more gradual and mild. In some cases there are no symptoms.

Acute back pain from a sudden compression fracture can last several weeks or months, and pain stemming from spinal deformity can persist indefinitely. For most, the severe pain subsides over a 6 to 12 week period as the vertebra is healing. Others suffer from pain long after the fracture has healed.

Often the symptoms of back pain from fracture are ignored or blamed instead on stress from daily activities, arthritis, or a natural progression of aging. If you experience any signs of fracture it is important to see a health care provider immediately to discuss these concerns. If diagnosed with a fracture, seek treatment at once to help avoid future fractures.

Humpback, Swayback, & Other Side Effects

The physical impacts of spinal fractures can be devastating. What begins for many as a loss in height may eventually lead to a humped back and other spinal deformities. Because of the shape and alignment of vertebrae and discs in the spine, several natural curves are formed that assist the body in movement and range of flexibility. The cervical spine (neck) and lumbar spine (lower back) have a normal inward curvature that is medically referred to as *lordosis*. The thoracic spine (upper back) has a normal outward curvature that is medically referred to as *kyphosis*. Multiple compression fractures can cause abnormal spinal curvatures such as excessive *lordosis,* an extreme inward curve in the lower back, also known as swayback, or excessive *kyphosis*, an extreme forward bend in the upper back. Another possible devastating side effect from compression fractures is *scoliosis*, a deformity where the spine bends to the left or right.

Figure 6.3: Normal (left) vs. Lordosis (middle) vs. Kyphosis (right)

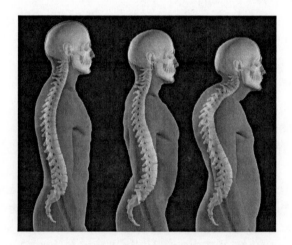

Figure 6.4: Normal Spinal Column (left) vs. Scoliosis (right)

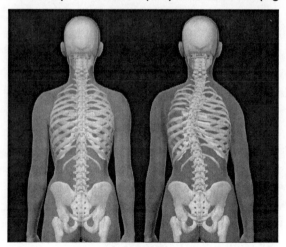

Possible physical impacts of spinal fractures are:

- Loss of height
- Ongoing acute pain
- Compressed internal organs
- Protruding abdomen
- Humpback
- Swayback
- Scoliosis
- Immobility
- Difficulty walking unaided
- Interference with breathing in cases where the rib cage presses down on the pelvis
- Limited flexibility and range of motion
- Heartburn
- Constipation
- Bowel obstruction
- Blood clotting.

A fracture in the vertebra can start out as a tiny crack and progress into something more severe. This can lead to instability in your spine—your tower of strength. It can disrupt and affect surrounding ligaments, muscles and discs. As the spine is designed to protect and support the body and organs, when a vertebra does break, the body's first response is to begin healing. Initially a granular material called a callus is formed at the fracture site. Collagen, a protein, is transported to the site through the blood stream. Collagen helps to mend and knit the fracture together. After new bone is joined with the old bone it is hardened through a process called calcification. Although your body begins to mend and heal the broken bone, you may be suffering from the consequences of the fracture.

The pain I experienced from vertebral fractures was worsened by the daily mental anguish and frustration of seeing no end in sight, of not knowing when or if ever I would be pain-free or return to a semi-normal life. I could only wish for a magic formula that would miraculously cure me. My physicians could prescribe, but not heal. I had to win this battle for myself.

Figure 6.5: Physical impact of spinal fractures

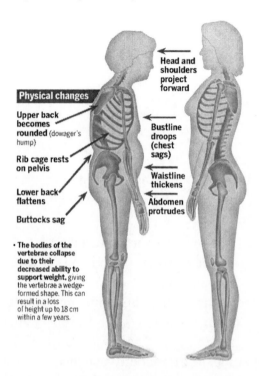

Physical changes

Upper back becomes rounded (dowager's hump)

Rib cage rests on pelvis

Lower back flattens

Buttocks sag

• The bodies of the vertebrae collapse due to their decreased ability to support weight, giving the vertebrae a wedge-formed shape. This can result in a loss of height up to 18 cm within a few years.

Head and shoulders project forward

Bustline droops (chest sags)

Waistline thickens

Abdomen protrudes

Fortunately, through determination and several months of research, I found a combination of therapies (along with various medications) that helped me reach my recovery goals:

- Bed rest
- Pain management
- Self-care
- Physical therapy
- Exercise
- Body mechanics and posture
- Bracing
- Surgical options
- Healing emotions
- Nutrition.

I hope you use and adapt the information shared in the following chapters to hasten your journey towards healthier bones and away from the risk of a devastating fracture.

CHAPTER 7

~

BED REST & THE ROAD
TO RECOVERY

After my spinal fractures, all I wanted to do was stay in bed. The least painful position for me was lying horizontal and staying motionless.

It is important to rest after a vertebral fracture as the body has suffered trauma—a broken bone—and it needs time to rest in order to heal. Bed rest can minimize the irritation in your spine and reduce local inflammation. Since inflammation can be one of the causes of your back pain, resting in the proper position can promote healing. However, staying in bed for more than a few days is not recommended (particularly for elderly patients) because the harm starts to outweigh the benefits. Although you may want to stay in bed—it is less painful and you worry less about causing new fractures—it is important to get up and get mobile. Remaining in bed for longer than 3 to 4 days can lead to:

- Weakening (atrophy) of muscles and ligaments

- Loss of fitness in your heart and lungs

- Stomach and bowel problems such as heartburn and constipation

- Circulation problems such as blood clots in the legs

- Further bone loss.

To begin recovery, it is essential to resume some form of normal activity as early as possible, no matter how difficult it is. It may hurt. In fact, from my experience, it will hurt. But our bones and muscles respond well to movement and activity and, in the long run, you will improve more quickly if you are able to ease back into your usual routine. Even though you may still feel pain, the idea is to take baby steps to regain strength and resume daily activities. It is difficult to fathom at the time—trust me—but the sooner you start moving again, the sooner your back pain will lessen. The ideal is to alternate between some form of activity and then rest throughout the day to gradually regain and build muscle and strength. I began with short walks around the house from the dining room to the kitchen, with assistance, and then gradually moved to short walks outside around the block. Then I made a point of rewarding myself by reading from a favourite magazine and enjoying a cup of coffee.

Practical Tips

Try not to be over ambitious (as I was a few times). If you increase your activity and the pain worsens—then cut back the next day.

Avoid falling back into the too-much-bed-rest trap by using your most comfortable and supportive chair as your daytime resting place between activities.

Now I Lay Me Down to Sleep

Getting a good night's sleep is essential to help your body and mind recover from the injury to your spine.

Prior to learning the proper mechanics of getting in and out of bed, lying in bed, and turning over in bed, what was supposed to be a time for relief and rest was more of a nightmare for me. After much pain and suffering I learned these practical tips through trial and error and my physiotherapist. In retrospect, I wish I had addressed the "sleeping" issue sooner, but my medical team and I were focused on other issues and I didn't understand how much of a difference a good night's sleep would make to my quality of life.

With a spinal fracture(s) the simple act of sleeping becomes a challenge. But relief is on the way! The key is to carry out simple movements, keep the spine aligned, and protect it from further injury. I suggest that you get a physiotherapist or occupational therapist to teach you how to get in and out of bed in a way that prevents further pain and/or injury. The following pages outline the sequence that I was taught in order to get in and out of bed without pain.

Getting Into Bed

It is tempting to flop into bed when you are tired but that twisting force on the spine is dangerous for someone with osteoporosis. These simple steps can ensure a safe way to settle in for the night:

1. Sit on the side of the bed.
2. Rest your arm closest to the pillow on the bed.
3. Lean toward the head of the bed keeping your head aligned with your spine.
4. Gradually let your body down by shifting your weight from your palm to your forearm, to your elbow, and then to your neck until you are lying down, bringing both legs up at the same time.
5. Then settle into a comfortable position.

Getting Out of Bed

(Never sit up straight from a lying position as this puts tremendous force on your spine):

1. Lie on your side facing the edge of the bed you are going to exit.
2. Bend your knees.
3. Ease yourself over to the edge of the bed.
4. While keeping the spine as straight as possible (no twisting), and using the arm closest to the bed, gradually push yourself up to a sitting position.
5. Place your hands on the bed behind you and push up to a standing position.

The optimum lying positions for most people to relieve stress on the back and keep the spine aligned are:

*   On your back with a pillow under your knees
*   On your back with both hips and knees bent with your legs propped up

- On your side with hips and knees bent and a pillow between your knees.

The pillow helps provide relief by taking some of the pressure off your spine. Avoid sleeping on your stomach as it puts pressure on the spine. For those who cannot get to sleep unless they are on their stomach, I suggest putting a pillow under the stomach to prevent the back from curving and creating pressure points on the spine.

To protect your spine in bed, keep it aligned when turning over. Avoid any twisting motion.

How to Turn Over in Bed—the Log Roll

1. Keep your shoulders aligned with your pelvis.
2. Extend your arms.
3. Bend your knees.
4. Slowly breathe in and gently pull in your abdominal muscles (if you can) and roll your whole body (log) over as a unit.

I still use these techniques today to minimize pain and strain on my spine.

The references and resources section at the back of this book includes valuable websites with diagrams and videos to help guide you through the important steps of getting into and out of bed as well as the log roll.

Practical Tip

Support your spine. Sitting or lying on soft surfaces that you sink into can be very painful for someone with spinal fractures. For myself, when I sit on couches that sink or soft bed mattresses it almost feels like the vertebrae in my spine are being squished together. It is most uncomfortable and sometimes downright painful, so I avoid it at all costs!

A firm (but not rock hard!) mattress and seats for your furniture is best. If you have a soft mattress or a sinking couch, it is well worth the investment to buy a new one. When you purchase couches and chairs you can specify the firmness of the foam.

My Diary

October 2001

After I had fractured my spine, but before I (or my doctors) realized that is what had happened, we did everything imaginable to try and get rid of the pain I felt. I tried massage therapy and physiotherapy at a private clinic that I had used previously for a knee injury. In hindsight this was not a good idea—they did not have a diagnosis and assumed it was back pain from the caesarian section. I left the treatments in more pain than when I arrived. I later learned that the exercises they gave me were harmful to my fractures, especially the pelvic tilt.

Many items were purchased to help my back, including a firmer mattress, two sturdy Lazy-Boy chairs, one of which included good lumbar support, heat, and massage. Bye-bye butter-soft leather couch!

Prior to my fracture diagnosis, and thinking my back pain would disappear in a week or two, my friends and family helped as caregivers for my daughter. But once we realized that my back was not progressing as expected, we hired a full-time caregiver who was a true blessing—I would say she nurtured both my daughter and I equally. She was an angel!

Nov 2001

The pain was chronic and overwhelming. I experienced physical pain as well as mental anguish because of my inability to take care of my one and only child. It hurt to sit, to stand, to lie down, and to even roll over in bed. One night I lay in bed in tears and realized something was drastically wrong. I knew this could not possibly be the normal back pain associated with a C-section.

As the pain reached an unbearable height, my husband and I went to Emergency. A doctor took x-rays and noted that my bones showed signs of being awfully thin on the x-rays for someone my age. He referred me to an orthopedic surgeon. The pain was continuous. It hurt to sit, stand, and lie down. I could not get relief. I told myself "I will get through this and then things will get better." The health care staff told me to be patient and that it takes time to see a specialist. In the mean time I was given stronger medication to ease the pain. I prayed each night that my back would get better and that the crippling pain would go away.

At my first appointment with an orthopedic surgeon who is a spine specialist he told me I had the muscles of someone 85 or older. Most likely due to the eight weeks of bed rest before the birth and the lack of mobility after my daughter was born. But he told me that we could create a plan to start recovery and build up the muscles. The doctor had many ambitious patients who were athletes. I told him my goal was to be able to take care of my daughter. He assured me that this was reasonable and manageable. Material things were no longer important; all I wanted was my health. I was an independent, energetic person and then after my back injury I could not be left alone with my own daughter as I was unable to lift her or feed her. I often whispered to my daughter, "Mommy can't do much right now but I will make up for it when I am well." I sometimes envied my caregiver, Doyet, as her bond with my daughter had become stronger than my own.

We arranged for an occupational therapist to visit our home to teach me new ways of performing all the things I used to do unthinkingly. I needed to learn how to do them safely and without further injury.

Then one day I received a phone call at home from my physician. A bone scan revealed five fractures—T11, T12, L1, L2 and L3. I didn't even know where these were exactly—just that there were five broken bones in my back! I was told that I had severe osteoporosis. I was relieved that there was a diagnosis but was overwhelmed by the reason and not sure what to do. I begged my physician to admit me into the hospital as I hoped for a quick solution to end the pain and misery and allow me to take care of my baby.

This was so difficult for my husband who had to manage everything: a new job, a new baby, and me. I worried about him being able to do it all for us and stay well.

I was admitted into hospital December 7, 2001 for five days. This allowed me to get procedures done over a few days in lieu of weeks or months including: x-rays, blood work, and a bone mineral density test.

I arrived home with a walker to get around on the main floor and a cane to get up the stairs. This felt very odd to me as I was used to going 100 mph. I realized more than ever that material possessions were meaningless without my health. I couldn't wait to be able to walk without aid and be able to carry my daughter. It was probably a good thing that I didn't know how much work I would need to do before I reached these previously simple goals!

Dec. 2001

Daylight was short and it was cold and icy so I was in the house most of the time. I worried that a slip could break more bones. I began to stay in bed longer each morning, take a longer nap each afternoon, and went to bed earlier each night. The pain was constant but seemed to diminish somewhat when lying down. If you break a bone in your leg or arm a cast is put on to allow the bone to heal. You can't really immobilize the spine to allow fractures to heal—a brace merely provides a bit of support. In addition, every move you make requires the help of your spine, whether it be sitting, standing, or lying down. Merely turning over in bed required me to brace myself, take a deep breath, and pull on the sheets or my husband to make and complete the turn.

All I wanted for Christmas was a strong, healthy back. Instead I received a shower bar, a railing for the front steps, and a treadmill!

Jan. 2002

I did my best to think positively and begin a journey of recovery. I tried to walk a little more each day with my walker whether I wanted to or not. The mornings were good. In the afternoons I was tired and sore. I was unable to shower without the help of my husband and getting dressed took a long time. I had lost a great deal of flexibility so I couldn't put my socks on without a "sock-aid." At first I thought it was the most ridiculous apparatus but then realized it gave me independence.

I made it around the block pushing my daughter in the jogger. It provided support. My caregiver Doyet and I were elated! I tried to be grateful and celebrate every improvement. Doyet, Chanel, and I ventured out shopping for the first time since my diagnosis!

It was difficult getting out in the winter so I made arrangements for a physiotherapist to come to the house. The rheumatologist I met in the hospital recommended her. She was very knowledgeable, compassionate, and disciplined. I trusted her. I wanted to ask her when I would get better but I was afraid of the answer. She provided me with incredibly useful tips to keep my spine aligned during daily activities, and the oh-so-important getting in and out of bed and how to turn over in bed. I do feel that meeting her was a turning point for me and it paved the way for my road to recovery.

Everyone's recovery rate from fracture and journey towards healthy bones will be different. But we all recover that much faster if we can find our way back to a good night's sleep.

CHAPTER 8

~

PAIN: WHAT IT IS, WHY IT HAPPENS & MEDICATION OPTIONS TO MANAGE IT

"Chronic pain is a thief. It breaks into your body and robs you blind. With lightning fingers, it can take away your livelihood, your marriage, your friends, your favourite pastimes and big chunks of your personality."

-Claudia Wallis, *Time* magazine, February 28, 2005

Pain can consume you. It can change your entire world. It can be relentless. Until I was diagnosed with five vertebral factures, I had no symptoms of osteoporosis, even though it develops over time (decades, even). What jolted me to its impact was the excruciating, debilitating constant pain just weeks after the birth of my daughter.

Writing this chapter brought back many horrible memories of living with searing pain and the struggle to get help to manage it. I tried several medications to manage my acute pain.

Pain was what actually alerted me to the fractures. I had always been able to manage minor aches and pains with Tylenol. When this did not diminish the pain at all I knew that something was terribly wrong with my back. The pain was severe and eventually led to me taking Tylenol with codeine for several months. I clearly remember waiting anxiously for the clock to arrive at the time when I could take my next pain pill. As the fractures healed and I became more mobile and began a series of stretches and exercises, I was able to wean myself off pain medication.

The one side effect from pain medication which no one likes to experience or talk about is constipation. It can become a real problem if you do not anticipate this and take steps to prevent it. As well as being uncomfortable, constipation can affect your appetite at a time when you need to help your body with good nutrition. Talk to your doctor about the option of taking stool softeners and increase your fibre and water intake to ensure your bowels don't come to a halt and your "conveyor belt" continues to run smoothly.

When I do strain my back and feel pain I assess it and decide whether I can manage it with rest, gentle stretches, and an over-the-counter pain medication or whether I need to see my doctor or physiotherapist (depending on how bad the pain is) to ensure that I have not sustained another fracture or serious injury.

Pain is hard to measure as it is a subjective experience. One person can never truly feel or understand another person's pain. Many are unaware of the options available to them to manage pain and regain their life. The decisions you take to manage your pain have the power to profoundly affect your health and your life. I encourage you to manage your pain assertively so you can lead a productive life. The idea is to present options that you can discuss with your health care team or a pain specialist. No one should suffer needlessly after fractures.

According to the National Institute of Health (US) a fractured vertebra can take anywhere from 6 to 8 weeks for the bone to set and up to 12 weeks to heal completely. But recovery from a vertebral fracture goes beyond healing the bone. Recovery becomes an ongoing process to regain strength and mobility and to resume your daily activities. Everyone experiences a slightly different recuperation. You may find your posture changing and have some nagging pain. This is because a vertebral fracture results in a deformity of the vertebra itself, which affects muscles, tendons, ligaments, and nerves near the fractured bone. When a vertebra is damaged, the spine makes adjustments to keep the body in balance, which may cause muscle pain. This pain can stop over time as the body adjusts to its new shape. Fortunately, if it does not, there are steps you can take to manage pain.

The spine is the center of well-being. When the vertebrae are damaged the consequence at the forefront of our minds is the pain—and how to get rid of it. The pain can range from mild to unbearable. After my fractures the pain was debilitating. It affected me in many ways. Everything hurt–even just lying in bed. It made me angry and anxious. I lost my appetite and steadily lost weight to the point of emaciation. I forgot what it was like to have a good night's sleep. The pain was a nightmare that I wanted to end. I could rarely sit for more than 20 minutes and could barely do anything without assistance. Being the type of person who can't stand to stay still, I would push myself to try to do too much. And even more so because I was a new mother. The result was exhaustion and increased pain.

Most books written about osteoporosis are written by health professionals rather than patients living with fractures. So they spend little time on the most debilitating consequences of spinal fracture—the searing pain. Most of the calls and e-mails I get are from women across North America struggling with their relentless, excruciating pain. And I know all too well the attitude of busy doctors towards patients who constantly chase them to get relief from chronic pain. Some feel that the patient is complaining unnecessarily and should suck it up, practice patience, and that in due course things will get better. Not an easy pill to swallow for a new mother who cannot even hold her baby because of her back pain!

Pain is often treated as an annoying side effect of spinal fractures. But pain is a four-letter word—nasty, powerful, and a serious health issue.

I want to help you take an active role in managing your pain—it is a huge part of reclaiming your life. To do so I will share my understanding of what pain is and how it affects us, tips on talking to your doctors about pain, and present some options to help you manage it.

Pain: What it Is & Why it Hurts

Pain is essential. Pain is the body's way of responding to an injury. It acts like a warning system to protect you from further injury. When a bone breaks, nerves send shrieking messages through the spinal cord to the brain, where they are interpreted. According to Dr. Augustus A. White III, author of *Your Aching Back*, your pain isn't actually at the point of injury (i.e., in your lower back). In a very real sense, it's in your brain. This is important because it means that pain can be controlled by preventing pain signals from reaching the brain. If the pain signals never reach the brain, you don't feel pain. This gives us a clue about how to deal with it. Pain is not just about an injury—it is about your brain's perception of that injury (the psychological factors affecting it).

Many athletes do not feel pain while they are competing. For example, if you are a runner in the midst of running a marathon and you trip or experience a minor injury, you may not experience any pain. Your pain "gates" may be closed because your brain is completely focused on something other than your symptoms at that moment in time. Once the marathon is complete you may suddenly begin to feel pain in the injured area. This suggests that a "gate" somewhere in the spinal cord slows or stops pain transmission by closing and increases it by opening.

Here is how the gate control theory works. In 1965 Professors Melazack and Wall suggested that there was a "gate" within the spinal cord which allowed messages to pass through to the brain. The theory states that nerve impulses, evoked by injury, are influenced in the spinal cord by other nerve cells that act like gates, either preventing the impulses from getting through, or facilitating their passage. In other words, the brain is not a passive receiver of pain information but can influence the information received, deciding whether it is important enough to be registered.

Whether the gate is open, closed, or partially closed depends on what sort of signal it receives from the brain. Emotions, expectations, prior experiences—even cultural attitudes—can play a part. When the gates are opening, pain messages get through more easily and pain can be intense. When the gates close, pain messages are prevented from reaching the brain and may not even be experienced. It is easier to understand with an example.

If you touch a hot stove, the nerves in the skin of your hand are vigorously stimulated, which causes impulses to race along the nerve fibers to the "gate" up the spinal cord to the brain. The brain then tells you about the pain and how you feel it. Once the nerve signal reaches the brain, the sensory information is processed in the context of your current mood, state of attention, and prior experience. The integration of all this information influences the perception and experience of pain, and guides your response.

The brain's response to this information will determine the extent of pain we get. If the brain sends a message back down to close the gate, the pain signals to the brain are blocked and we experience lower pain. (That message may be carried by endorphins, natural painkillers in the body that are chemically similar to morphine.) If the brain orders the pain gates to open wider, the pain signal intensifies, sometimes to the point of debilitation. For example, assume a mother and daughter are cooking together and an accident in the kitchen leads to boiling water being spilled on both of them. The mother is so worried about the child that she doesn't feel the pain of the burn. The concern for her child has caused the natural release of endorphins, which block the pain signal and prevent her from noticing the pain.

Although no one yet truly understands the details of this process or how to control it, the following concepts are presented to help explain why various treatments are effective and how to find solutions to back pain after spinal fractures.

The same "gate" principles apply in back pain. The nerve endings that detect pain are present in many structures in the back, including the muscles and ligaments, the disks, the vertebrae, and the facet joints. When one of these parts is irritated or mechanically malfunctioning the pain message will be transmitted by special peripheral nerves to the spinal cord and up to the brain. These messages can be over-ridden by other signals produced by the various treatments which will be discussed in this chapter and Chapters 9 to 17.

Non-surgical ways to close your pain gates include but are not limited to: heat and ice massage, regular massage, and acupuncture—these probably send stimuli to the brain telling it to close the pain gates. The common denominator of all these methods is that they interrupt pain messages between the back and the brain.

Drugs such as muscle relaxants, for example, can block pain messages. Our bodies produce their own painkillers, called endorphins. Different mechanisms can stimulate the brain to produce endorphins. Acupuncture and relaxation techniques such as meditation and hypnosis may lead to the production of endorphins and help dull pain.

Anxiety, depression, and other negative emotions can intensify pain, either lowering the threshold for pain sensitivity or altering the brain's interpretation of it. One reason chronic pain is so hard to resolve is that the memory of pain tends to lower your pain threshold, resulting in a more intense response.

Short-term & Long-term Pain—Acute & Chronic Pain

We tend to have a pretty simplistic view of pain, including many health care professionals. Pain to us often means a part of the body is damaged. And pain hurts. So, if you are like me, you want relief. Now! However, I now know that it is not quite as simple as it appears. Understanding the pain you are experiencing can be the first step to relief. Get to know your body in terms of how it is dealing with the injury—in this case one or more spinal fractures. Then you can choose the best approaches to manage your individual pain. Pain intensity and relief varies among people with fractures. And I can attest to the fact that unrelieved pain, whether it is short-term or long-term, can have both negative physical and psychological consequences. Pain is generally divided into two categories: acute and chronic.

Acute Pain

Acute back pain can be the first symptom of a spinal fracture. The pain may be described as sharp, nagging, or dull; and movement may exacerbate the pain. Acute pain is short-term, lasting anywhere from a few hours to six months and can be cured or managed. It is our body's way of warning us that something in our body has been injured and to be cautious so as to prevent further injury. After a vertebral fracture the pain can be fast and somewhat sharp and then it can be followed by longer-term aching pain in and around the fracture. In my case the pain was constant and severe enough that it resulted in a five day hospital stay.

Osteoporosis can cause very painful fractures. In many cases the pain starts to subside as the fracture heals. Most fractures heal within three months. Some people experience pain for a short time after a fracture and it disappears gradually within 12 weeks. Others continue to have muscle spasms and pain, particularly with prolonged standing or walking, after the fracture is healed. Muscle spasms are involuntary contractions of a muscle. A spasm feels like tightness or a knot in a muscle. People can have "tight" muscles in their back near the fracture and may find that the muscles hurt and are difficult to use. The pain eases once the muscle gradually relaxes. Acute pain usually responds well to medications.

Chronic Pain

One in six North Americans suffer from chronic or recurrent pain (Claudia Willis, *Time Magazine* Feb. 28, 2005). Many are in misery and don't quite understand why or how to get relief. Chronic pain interferes with leading a normal life, both physical and emotional. Another very important step toward getting better after a fracture is to understand what chronic pain is. Our common understanding of pain is that it tells us when we have damaged our body. We need pain so that we can tell when we are injuring ourselves. However this simplistic view of pain does not explain why, once your fracture has healed and your doctor has not found any new injury, you still have pain.

Chronic pain often occurs daily and persists or recurs for more than six months (or beyond the point the fracture has healed). It is no longer a help but a hindrance, as the body no longer needs a code red alert to prevent further injury.

In chronic pain the nervous system may be sending a pain signal even though there is no ongoing damage in your spine. It can be affected by many things including your state of mind, your thoughts, your overall health, and your emotional well-being (depression, anxiety, etc.). For example, when angry or anxious—and it is tough not to feel anxious after a fracture—your pain can feel more intense.

Some people with vertebral fractures live with varying degrees of chronic or recurrent pain. They may have good days where the pain is minimal and other days when it can be quite severe. The fracture has healed but the pain continues. It may be triggered by muscle spasms, stiffness, poor body mechanics, or muscle fatigue.

I live with recurrent pain. Some days I know I have irritated my back by doing something incorrectly while exercising or during my daily activities. I might lift an object without being cautious and the resulting twist to my spine triggers the pain. I do my best to be careful, but nobody is perfect.

In chronic pain the nervous system may be sending a pain signal even though there is no ongoing damage to the spine. The nervous system itself misfires and creates the pain. It is almost as though a chemical switch has been turned on and won't turn off. This could be due to the fact that there are naturally occurring chemicals used by our nervous system to transmit pain messages. These chemicals are called neurotransmitters and there are many different types. Some of these neurotransmitters can help decrease pain. There are other neurotransmitters that may increase pain.

One theory is that the nervous system has an imbalance of these naturally occurring neurotransmitters. The ones that decrease pain do not seem to be working as well—and the ones that increase pain seem to be in overdrive. In these situations, the pain message being sent does not signify that something is being damaged or is about to be damaged. Thus it is not a useful message for us and the system is not working the way it should.

Chronic pain, although often more challenging to treat than acute pain, can be managed and you can lead an active life. Because chronic pain can be influenced by such things as lack of exercise, your thoughts about the pain, and emotional states such as depression and anxiety it is important to identify what factors may be contributing to your pain.

Pain should not be ignored. Left untreated it can lead to depression, loss of muscle, sexual dysfunction, heartburn, bowel problems, insomnia, and isolation from friends and family. You would be a rare individual if you did not experience periods of frustration, anger, and even depression when living with chronic pain. Please read on because there are things that can be done to alleviate your suffering.

Enough about pain, let's move on to how you can find relief.

Categorizing pain is important because it helps doctors determine the best way of treating pain. A treatment that works on one type of pain will not necessarily be appropriate for another type of pain. So the first step in any treatment plan is to determine what type of pain you are dealing with. Use the following steps when talking to your doctor about your pain (it may be helpful to write it out in advance, as it can be difficult to remember everything you want to bring up during the visit):

1. Rate your pain on a scale from 1 to 10, with 10 being the highest.

2. Describe the type of pain—sharp, nagging, dull, intense, throbbing, intermittent, constant, etc.

3. Share where your pain is located.

4. Describe what movements increase your pain.

5. Explain how pain is affecting your life—limiting daily activities, withdrawal from family and friends, anxiety, depression, economically, etc. Don't minimize the consequences.

6. Provide a list of the medications you take, in what dosages, and how often.

7. Share what is relieving your pain, whether treatment, rest, certain positions, or medication.

Doctors often have a tough time with chronic pain because it is hard to diagnose the cause and finding solutions is time consuming. If you don't make your pain a priority, it is unlikely that your doctor will do so.

What Can I Do to Relieve My Back Pain?

There are many options. The first thing I would suggest is you put all your assumptions aside. You will need to stop looking for a single solution to relieving your pain. Instead, I suggest you examine a combination of different approaches and treatments that complement each other. Some of the treatments you have tried before that did not work may help when combined with a different combination of therapies. There are many things you can do to help yourself. Explore options and you can discover what works best for you.

Both drug and non-drug treatments can be successful in helping to prevent and control pain. You can talk to your health care team/ doctor and decide which ones are best for you. Many people combine two or more methods (outlined in Chapters 9 to 17) to get relief.

Barriers to Seeking Pain Relief (from Spineuniverse.com)

Many people with chronic pain don't seek pain relief, or even tell their doctors about their pain. The Spineuniverse.com site nicely sums up the more common reasons:

- Fear of being labeled as a "bad patient." You won't find relief if you don't talk with your doctor about the pain you feel

- Fear that increased pain may mean that the disease has worsened. Regardless of the state of your disease, the right treatment for pain may improve daily life for you and your family

- Fear of addiction to drugs. Research has shown that the chance of people with chronic pain becoming addicted to pain-relieving drugs is extremely small. When taken properly for pain, drugs can relieve pain without addiction. Needing to take medication to control your pain is not addiction

- Lack of awareness about pain therapy options. Be honest about how your pain feels and how it affects your life. Ask your doctor about the pain therapy options available to you. Often, if one therapy isn't effectively controlling your pain, another therapy can. New medications and pain relief techniques are constantly being developed

- Fear of being perceived as "weak." Some believe that living stoically with pain is a sign of strength, while seeking help often is considered negative or weak. This perception prevents them seeking the best treatment with available therapies.

Don't let fears and misconceptions keep you from talking to your doctor and other members of your health care team about getting adequate pain relief. Help and relief are possible, but only if you discuss your symptoms with your doctor.

Medications & Feeling Better

Most people have taken some form of pain medication to ease pain, whether for something as simple as a headache or for a more serious injury such as a sprain. The majority of pain medication is designed to help manage shorter-term acute pain. However, pain medication may be prescribed for longer time periods (a year or even longer). Although many people do not want to be on pain medication, they often accept this option to help them manage the pain and ease recovery—for some recovery would be almost impossible without relief from constant pain.

People recover more quickly when pain is better managed or—even better—fully relieved. So the goal is to take the medication that works best to alleviate your pain, thereby allowing you to improve your ability to be mobile and perform daily tasks, then to get the necessary therapy, and finally to come off the medication. All current medications have their limitations and possible side effects, especially when taken for prolonged periods of time.

Pain Medication Options

Consulting with your doctor is critical to find a pain medication that works for you. I define a working medication as one that alleviates or diminishes the pain and does not cause unwanted complications. It is important to report back to your doctor if you have any side effects from the pain medication(s) you are taking. It is also helpful to consult with your pharmacist on the best time of day and means to take the medication.

It is important to remember that drugs are not a cure. They help minimize the pain but they do not heal the fracture. The one exception is anti-inflammatories which can help lessen the soft-tissue damage by reducing the swelling. My experience was that drugs minimized the pain but never fully removed it. I suppose this is a good thing for if we completely mask all pain we can take on too much activity too quickly and cause more physical damage.

You and your doctor may decide on an over-the-counter pain reliever and then, if the pain is still not manageable, request a prescription for a stronger medication. These interventions may not eliminate your pain completely, but hopefully you will find enough relief to become more active and do the things that you enjoyed pre-fracture.

Prior to popping any pills, I urge you to review and discuss the options that follow over the next pages with your physician (and possibly your pharmacist) to choose a pain medication that it is right for you. It is essential to look at your medical history, other medications you are taking, and the need to balance pain relief with potentially adverse side effects. Then pick whatever works best—you may not care about why it works!

The following sections describe the most commonly used pain relief medications, how they work, why they might be prescribed to you, and possible side effects.

The Big Four (most commonly used pain medications)

1. Non-Steroidal Anti-Inflammatory Drugs (NSAIDs)

The most common are aspirin (e.g., Bayer Aspirin, Anacin), and Ibuprofen (e.g., Advil, Motrin). They help reduce pain and swelling by blocking our cells from releasing the chemicals that cause inflammation and trigger transmission of pain signals to the brain. They are considered quite safe, are effective, inexpensive, and can be mostly obtained without a prescription (stronger forms like Aleve may require a prescription in some jurisdictions).

The main possible side effect of the NSAID class of medication is stomach problems, such as an upset stomach, indigestion and, more rarely, ulcers (with or without bleeding). Certain risk factors can create a higher likelihood of heart attack or stroke in some patients. They can also be hard on your liver and kidneys. Naproxen and Ibuprofen may have gastrointestinal side effects. NSAIDs can intensify or, alternatively, counteract the effects of some medications. The risk and severity of the side effects increase the longer you take NSAIDs.

2. Acetaminophen

It is most commonly known by the brand name Tylenol and works by elevating the body's overall pain threshold so that you feel less pain—it reduces pain, but not inflammation. It is less likely than NSAIDs to irritate the stomach. Some doctors will suggest both acetaminophen and an anti-inflammatory in an effort to control pain. Acetaminophen does not require a prescription and has almost no side effects, although too-high doses can create serious damage to the liver.

3. Muscle Relaxants

This class of drugs blocks the nerve signals from the brain and spinal cord that cause muscles to contract and spasm. Brand names include Robax Platinum and Robaxet and manufacturers often combine a muscle relaxant and a pain reliever.

Doctors seem to have mixed feelings about muscle relaxants. They do not heal the injury, but they can help muscles relax and hence ease your discomfort. Proponents of muscle relaxants believe that reducing the intensity of a muscle spasm will reduce the pain. Other physicians are unsure as to whether the relaxants effectively target the muscles that are in spasm. It is not known if they act directly on the target muscles or act centrally in the brain and function as more of a general body relaxant. Many doctors prefer to prescribe them only if a severe muscle spasm is not responding to anti-inflammatories or other medications.

Because a muscle relaxant may lead you to feel as if your injury is healed, it can be tempting to resume normal activities, leading to further injury. Side effects include drowsiness (bad for driving!), dizziness (possible falls and further fracture), and they can be toxic to the liver.

4. Narcotic Analgesics

These are also known as pain killers, and include morphine, Demerol, codeine, and even medical heroin. They are used to treat moderate to severe pain. This class of medications affects the central nervous system and reduces sensitivity to pain by blocking the chemical receptors in the brain that sense pain. They do not heal the injury, they simply stop your perception of the pain. If your pain is severe and has not responded to other pain relievers, your physician may prescribe a narcotic analgesic (the word narcotic comes for the Ancient Greek *narkos*, "to numb"). Because it is so strong and has serious potential side effects, it is available by prescription only.

Side effects include dizziness, fatigue, impaired concentration, blurred vision and nausea. Constipation can also become a problem, particularly with codeine. They can become physically and psychologically addictive. Prolonged use causes the body to develop a tolerance, requiring higher dosages for the same pain numbing effect. Too high a dose can slow down or even stop breathing, resulting in death.

Other Pain Medication Options

Less common options to help patients with pain include, calcitonin, pain patches and epidural steroid injections. These are usually brought into play when the more common options have not delivered the hoped-for results.

Calcitonin

Calcitonin is primarily prescribed by doctors to regulate calcium and help reduce bone turnover by suppressing the activity of the osteoblasts. However, it has proven to be effective for some people to relieve pain from vertebral fractures. I discuss calcitonin in more detail in Chapter 17.

Pain Patch

Similar to a nicotine patch, a pain patch delivers pain medication gradually through the skin into the bloodstream. It delivers a powerful narcotic pain killer that can provide long-lasting relief from persistent severe to moderate pain. It can relieve pain for up to three days and is an option for those who require strong pain medication but are unable to tolerate swallowing pills or an intravenous pump. But the patch's effect can wear off before the 72 hours it is designed to last, and a new one can only be applied every 72 hours—resulting in the onset of pain.

This should only be used when other medicines are not effective and pain needs to be controlled around the clock. For example, a severe fall at the age of 89 caused my father to suffer spinal fractures and subsequent severe pain. His doctors decided that a pain patch would give him the best pain relief and least amount of stress.

As with many medications there can be serious side effects with the pain patch. Because of the risk of death from respiratory depression (difficulty breathing), the patch is only suitable for patients who are already tolerant to opioid therapy. As with all narcotics, addiction can be a risk for some patients. Unpleasant withdrawal symptoms may result if the medication must be stopped suddenly. Sleepiness, a sense of being sedated, and constipation are also common side effects. In the US there have been recalls and lawsuits due to manufacturing defects which led to the active drug leaking into the skin at an uncontrolled rate, causing breathing difficulties and even death.

Epidural Steroid Injections

A steroid injection (by a doctor) into the space around the spinal cord, called the epidural space, is referred to as an epidural steroid injection. They are not considered permanent pain fixes, but they are used to treat severe back pain and may last from one week up to one year. They are said to be successful because the medication is administered directly to the site of the problem. Epidural steroid injection is an outpatient procedure. As with all invasive medical procedures, there are potential risks associated with injections into the lower spine. In addition to temporary numbness of the bowels and bladder, the most common potential risks and complications include: infection, severe spinal headache, bleeding, and nerve damage.

Drugs—Are They the Answer?

Drugs are not a cure. The purpose of the pain medication is to try to allow you enough comfort to enjoy a good night's sleep in a comfortable position—not to get up and function fully without pain. You don't want to do too much and then cause more damage. You can become physically and psychologically dependent on drugs. Once you start healing and the pain gradually subsides, you will want to stop taking them or risk becoming reliant.

Some people with back pain can't move, can't function, and can't focus on anything but the pain—medications can help them get through this. Most family practitioners are willing to try just about anything that works for you—they want you to get some relief. But family physicians are not back specialists—so it can be frustrating for both of you as they try to get to the bottom of your back pain. Like headaches, back pain can be very challenging to treat. The idea is to weigh the relief medication brings against the risks it carries and figure out what dosages and timing bring the most benefits. For example, one very strong dosage at night may allow you to sleep well and get up and function the next day. But this same dosage may be too strong to use during the day because of drowsiness, dizziness, etc.

Back pain is very challenging to treat. It is sometimes difficult to determine why, after a fracture has healed, one patient still has recurring back pain and another does not. Most get relief after 3 to 6 months on their own or through some form of conservative treatment. Unfortunately, a small percentage of patients experience chronic back pain while others experience recurring back pain.

For myself, it comes and goes. I am cautious with my movements, exercise and stretch regularly, and am very conscious of best practices. I learned to say "No!" to many activities that, before my fractures, I saw as risk-free When I am tired I know that I am more prone to injury. But despite my efforts, I sometimes wake up with back pain—not really knowing how I irritated my spine again! People who are in good health and exercise regularly tend to get better faster than people who are not in good shape. For some, the back pain continues long after the fracture has healed. It just won't quit hurting. It can affect your life; it can affect your family; it can affect your work; it can affect your personality. It can be overwhelming and sometimes a person does not know where to turn for help—or is simply too tired and in too much pain to have the energy for yet another round of appointments.

Norma's Story

Norma, in her 70s, began corresponding with me by e-mail in 2008 after reading an article on me that appeared in newspapers across Canada. She had suffered debilitating pain from multiple compression fractures. "Since my first e-mail to you I am now free of the morphine and just take a Tylenol 3 if and when necessary. The pain I endured for the three weeks following the last of the morphine was worse than the back pain. Every single joint and muscle in my shoulders, knees, hips, wrists and hands was extremely painful on movement of any sort. The two months it took to wean myself off was bad enough, with flu like symptoms plus the sore joints and muscles progressively getting worse every day and then the last three weeks of it I was getting darned close to not wanting to even get up in the mornings. A good night's sleep has also escaped me since starting to get drug free but that I can deal with. Like you, bed was the one place I didn't hurt but that all changed when I started to drop the drug... even my bottom hurt if I was in bed for more than 4 to 6 hours. My hands were too painful to move the covers. The pain in the joints is now slowly subsiding and I can close my hands to make a fist in the morning (too swollen before). This week has been my best yet."

When it comes to pain after fracture, there is no quick solution or magic answer. However, there are options to choose from. If you know your options you can draw upon many sources to formulate your own plan to reduce or even eliminate pain. Drugs can help temporarily but non-drug treatments can be extremely effective at overpowering your pain. As Claudia Willis said "It takes more than a prescription pad to really bring pain relief" (*Time Magazine* Feb. 28, 2005) so let's move on and see what might work for you.

CHAPTER 9

~

SELF-CARE: THE SISTERS ARE DOING IT FOR THEMSELVES!

After being diagnosed with a spinal fracture or fractures, you have decisions to make—some big and some smaller—in terms of how they will impact you and your health in the short and long-term. The information in this chapter will help you work in partnership with your health care team. Appointments with health professionals are usually short and concise. The rest of the time it is you, your fractures, pain, and anxiety as you wonder if you will ever get your life back. It is important to know that once you get home from these appointments there are things that you can do that can help you alleviate pain and promote healing. For me, day-to-day pain management and some actions and treatments that soothed my body and soul were key parts of my overall recovery.

Some of the options I explored fell outside conventional Western medicine. Complementary therapies include mind-body therapies, in which the power of the mind or the spirit is harnessed to heal the body. They also encompass touch therapies, which involve massage and other forms of physical manipulation performed by practitioners to promote healing.

I found it helpful to keep an open mind and I urge you to consider a therapy you may not have been willing to try before. But be sure to consult with your doctor and other health care team members before beginning any complementary or alternative therapy.

Therapies to Care for Your Back Pain
Ice Therapy

An ice pack, applied to the painful areas, is a quick, simple, low risk, and inexpensive therapy to relieve pain, especially recurring pain. You can use ice in a bag, frozen vegetables like peas or corn, or a commercial gel ice pack. The cold of the ice narrows blood vessels, which helps slow down painful inflammation and tissue damage. It also slows down the nerves transmitting pain impulses to the brain, possibly even closing the "pain gate." It can help break the cycle of painful muscle spasms. Once the cold pack is removed, blood rushes into the injured area with the nutrients that help heal the injury.

Use the ice pack three times a day, but no more than 20 minutes each time. Do not apply ice directly to your skin—it should be contained in a bag, or wrapped in a cloth (towel, old t-shirt, etc.). Do not fall asleep with the ice pack. Anyone with Raynaud's disorder (blood flow disorder) or rheumatoid arthritis should not use an ice pack.

Talk to your doctor and physiotherapist to find out what regime will work best for you. Some people like to ice soon after the injury and then switch to heat therapy, others find that alternating between the two blocks pain more effectively. It may be necessary to experiment a little to find what works best for your body and pain.

Heat Therapy

The application of moist or dry heat is another low risk, inexpensive, and simple way to alleviate pain. A heat pack (gel) or a heat wrap (granules) can be applied for 20-60 minutes at a time. It is important not to overheat your hot pack, as you can burn your skin (and, because of the deeper pain, you may not be able to sense the damage being done to your skin until it is too late).

If you have access and sufficient mobility, a hot tub can be helpful with pain and generally relaxing—consult your doctor for the best temperature and suggested amount of time. Generally, 102 degrees Fahrenheit (39 C) is considered optimal and anything over 104 degrees (40 C) can lead to stroke, heart attack, and even brain damage.

Heat therapy works by expanding the blood vessels that surround the spine. This extra circulation carries away metabolic irritants and brings oxygen and nutrients to damaged tissues, promoting healing. Heat also stimulates the sensory receptors in the skin which decreases the transmission of pain signals to the brain. Just like cold therapy, it can close the "pain gate" and help break the cycle of muscle spasms which cause more pain. Heat relieves stiffness in soft tissue, allowing for more flexibility.

Most people can use heat therapy regularly without side effects, as long as temperature guidelines are adhered to. Heat therapy should not be used by anyone with diabetes, deep vein thrombosis, and dermatitis. Do talk to your doctor and physiotherapist for guidance, tips, and limitations that your specific medical history may require.

Massage Therapy

A massage therapist uses basic hand movements to apply pressure to the body's soft tissue (skin, muscles, tendons, and ligaments). Massage relieves pain, reduces stress, and promotes healing by improving circulation, deepening relaxation, and providing positive physical awareness and emotional well-being. It decreases painful muscle spasms, stimulates the nerves, and stretches and loosens muscles to keep them elastic, all of which may help close the brain's "pain gate."

In addition to helping with circulation and range of motion, massage may raise endorphin levels (the chemicals which make us feel good), reducing anxiety and depression, improving sleep, and lessening pain (although it may not help with inflammation). Massage therapy is thought to stimulate the parasympathetic nervous system, slowing down the heart and relaxing the body.

To prevent further injury, make sure that the massage therapist you work with is knowledgeable about osteoporosis and fractures. It is vital to share your medical history with your massage therapist. If you are homebound, licensed, reputable therapists are available for home visits. Massage is a general term that covers several methods such as Swedish, Shiatsu, trigger point, neuromuscular, etc. Consult with your doctor and/or physiotherapist as to which form of therapy will best suit your situation and ask if they can provide a referral.

Check your insurance coverage to see whether massage therapy is covered. If it is, you will probably need to get a referral from your doctor before starting your massage therapy in order to be reimbursed by the insurance company.

Alternative Approaches to Managing Long-Term Pain/Chronic Pain

Therapies that used to be considered "out there" have become more accepted over the past few decades (some insurers now cover the cost of acupuncture and hypnosis treatments, for example). While there is no firm explanation as to how these therapies work, there is plenty of anecdotal evidence that some people do find relief from pain by using them. The pain that I felt after my fractures brought a willingness to try anything that might help reduce the pain, as long as there was no risk of further damage.

If you decide to try alternate therapies, talk to your doctors and physiotherapists first. They may be able to recommend someone who is familiar with osteoporosis or know of another patient who will be willing to share their experience with the therapy and whether it relieved pain or stress. Be sure that alternate practitioners are experienced in treating people with osteoporosis and fractures and share your medical history with them. Check to see if their profession has a professional association and licensing body and if they are members in good standing. If the practitioner discourages you from talking to other patients, I would choose a different one. Relatively few serious adverse side effects have been reported for these treatments so they can be used over the long-term if you find them of benefit. Of course, the quality of the treatment will depend completely upon the experience and expertise of the service provider.

Acupuncture

Acupuncture comes from traditional Chinese medicine, where good health depends upon two things:

- The unobstructed flow of energy (*qi* or *chi)* through the body's 12 major channels (meridians)

- A balance between the hot (*yang*) and cool (*yin*) life force.

Illness and pain is believed to occur when the flow of *qi* is blocked or one when one life force dominates the other. Acupuncturists insert extremely thin needles into points along the meridians (thought to coincide with different parts of the body and organ systems) to redirect or unblock stagnant *qi*. Western science theorizes that acupuncture may stimulate large diameter nerve fibers that direct the brain to close the "pain gates" and/or release naturally occurring brain chemicals that reduce pain. Still others theorize that it has a strong placebo effect (which is known to be effective in pain mitigation). Because acupuncture does seem to provide some pain relief and it has no harmful side effects, it is gaining in popularity.

If you decide to try acupuncture, be sure to find a qualified practitioner—ask your doctor or physiotherapist if they are aware of and feel comfortable suggesting someone and use national acupuncture organizations as a resource. The Chinese Medicine & Acupuncture Society of Canada recommends that people with diseases like osteoporosis visit a fully qualified doctor of traditional Chinese medicine (TCMD), preferably one who has extensive clinical experience relating to osteoporosis. Also, the US National Centre for Complimentary and Alternative Medicine advises not to rely on a diagnosis of disease by an acupuncture practitioner who does not have substantial conventional medical training. Regulations regarding acupuncture vary widely between individual provinces and states. Get clear information about the course of treatment and how much it will cost. Be aware that any herbs that are suggested may interact for the worse with your prescribed medications.

Reiki

Reiki is a traditional Japanese technique for stress reduction and relaxation that is said to promote healing. It is also based on the idea of an unseen life force that causes us to feel poorly when it is low and happy and healthy when it is high. "Reiki" is a combination of two words, "rei" meaning "God's Wisdom" and "ki" which means "Life force energy." Literally, the word means "spiritually guided life force energy."

According to Tara Taylor, a reputable reiki master practicing in Calgary, reiki is a system of natural healing involving the "laying on of hands." It is not a massage. During a reiki treatment, the practitioner places their hands in a number of positions above or on the client's body, sending healing universal life energy wherever it needs to go in the body. Reiki helps to break up energy blockages within the body, allowing healing energy to flow again freely while stimulating the body's natural ability to heal itself on a physical, emotional, mental and spiritual level.

The client typically wears loose clothing and receives the treatment lying down. The reiki energy is perceived as heat coming from the practitioner's hands. It is said to gently stimulate the body's own innate wisdom to cure the cause of the problem. Although spiritual in nature, it is not part of a religion. Some people who receive it report feeling a wonderful, glowing radiance flowing around them and through them. Reiki practitioners' training and expertise vary. Increasingly, many people who seek training are licensed health care professionals. However, no licensing or professional standards exist for the practice of reiki in Canada or the US which is why talking to your doctor and other patients can give you valuable insights.

Hypnotherapy

Many of us automatically think of the entertainment industry when we hear the word hypnosis—volunteers on a stage acting in strange, uncontrolled ways. In the healing context, hypnosis applies subconscious suggestion to the mind of the patient. The client is brought into a deep state of relaxation (the brainwaves are slowed to alpha state) and then the mind is told how to respond to pain messages (lessening the perception of pain). Relaxation of the mind also affects the body, reducing painful muscle spasms in the back.

Hypnosis can help with back pain. By influencing the mind's perception of pain, it means that even though the pain signal is still there, your mind is giving it less attention, reducing (or even stopping) your sense of pain. It can also elevate your natural feel-good chemicals (endorphins) that anesthetize the damaged area. Finally, hypnosis can be used to help uncover emotional issues which elevate stress and can flood the body with chemicals that create inflammation and tightness, leading to muscle spasms. Pain has a real physical cause, but it can be worsened by your emotional state—and most of us naturally feel negative emotions after fractures. Hypnosis can help reduce or even eliminate both new and old emotional trauma.

People can learn and use self-hypnosis techniques to relax and reduce their pain. Many of the self-help regimes used to improve health, knowledge, and performance are forms of self-hypnosis. Repeating the desired suggestion constantly in the conscious mind will instill it in the unconscious.

Some people are so responsive to hypnosis that they can completely block their perception of pain. It is important to be aware that pain is sometimes giving you a message that something is wrong (perhaps your fracture has not healed or there is a new injury). It is not wise to eliminate the pain without discovering the cause. For this reason, it is important to seek a diagnosis of the cause from your doctor before dealing with the pain.

Buyer beware. One can actually learn the techniques to induce hypnosis in a weekend course. This does not make the person a professional. Most provinces and states exert little or no regulation over the practice of hypnosis.

Other Self-Care Suggestions

- Put your pride aside and be open to options that you may not have considered before that may help ease the pain and allow you to enjoy life

- Consider investing in an Obus Forme backrest support to ease pain and make sitting more comfortable at home, in the car, and when travelling. This product has an s-shape frame that molds your spine into proper anatomical alignment. It is specifically designed to enhance people's lives by decreasing pressure on the back and increasing comfort while sitting. It has provided much relief and comfort for many people that I know that have back pain. Some also find the Obus Forme seat helpful as it encourages proper alignment of the pelvis and thighs

- When purchasing your next vehicle, pay close attention to the comfort of the ride over bumpy roads (the suspension) and the car seats. Many sport utility vehicles are built on a truck chassis and can be unbearably rough, especially if you are in pain. People often think of the need for ergonomic seats in the home or office but fail to think of it when driving. And car seats, even in luxury cars, are not all ergonomic and are uncomfortable for people with back problems—especially those seats that are sporty, low, and curved. When buying a car, the seat is the most ergonomically important aspect to your ability to feel comfortable when you drive so be sure that all parts of it provide you with decent support and that all its adjustment controls can be operated easily by electronic mechanisms. Ensure that it is suitable in relation to your legs, hips, and back in particular as car seats come in all different shapes and sizes.

I use a number of options that complement what my health care team offers to stay well and help manage pain and stiffness. I have used ice at times to ease my back pain, especially in the hot summer months. I have to confess that I find a heat wrap is much more soothing to my soul. It helps ease stiffness and improves my flexibility, especially in the evenings of the cold winter months. Prior to my fractures, I used to love a warm, relaxing bath but now I find it challenging (even scary) to get in and out of the tub and it is uncomfortable sitting in the tub. I stick to warm showers instead. I do enjoy hot tubs and find them soothing.

I treat myself for a massage periodically with a therapist who I trust. I find it helps reduce muscle tension, aids my relaxation, and increases my flexibility. Lying on my back while the therapist works on my shoulders and neck proved to be uncomfortable until my therapist came up with a solution—slipping a warm heating pad under my back helps tremendously.

It is gratifying to find options and tools that bring not only a sense of relief but a feeling of control and independence. Some days, one option works better than another day. If nothing seems to work, talk to your doctor, who may refer you to a pain management program that suggests other ways to cope with long-term pain.

I use an Obus Forme daily at home and as added support in the car. When we purchased our last vehicle we told the salesperson that comfort was of utmost importance due to my back injury. He recommended the Toyota Avalon which we purchased and we are absolutely thrilled with its smooth ride!

As you can see, there are ways you can reduce and possibly even eliminate your pain. Your own initiatives will help greatly, but, as the following chapter shares, there are people you should add to your health care team who will help you make huge strides in reducing pain and living well with osteoporosis.

CHAPTER 10

~

PHYSICAL THERAPY: HELPING YOUR BODY HELP ITSELF

P hysical therapy is my lifeline.

A competent physiotherapist or osteopathic manual practitioner and an occupational therapist who are knowledgeable about osteoporosis can get you back into the game of life and moving again after fractures. It will not happen overnight—but it will happen! With patient commitment and guidance from both therapists you can maximize your motion, regain your strength and flexibility, and learn how to prevent further injury.

Every member of your health care team is important and interdependent. Your physician, your rheumatologist or endocrinologist, and your orthopedic surgeon will diagnose your disease and bone fractures as well as look at how to best manage and treat you in the short and long-term. They may prescribe medication. You may see each of these health care practitioners every six months or so, but you should see your physiotherapist weekly—or more.

In my view, your physiotherapist (PT) or osteopathic manual practitioner (OMP) and your occupational therapist (OT) are key partners that not only help you move again, but also help you regain confidence and the ability to better mange the disease. I cannot emphasize this enough. A good PT or OMP helps you better understand how your body has been impacted by the fractures, and learn how to listen to your body and help it heal. A good OT will help you learn new ways of doing things (e.g., lifting) and help improve your strength and abilities.

To better understand why and how these health professionals should be a part of your team I will share my understanding of their professions, what you can do, and what to watch out for.

Physiotherapy
What Is It?

Physiotherapy uses physical means such as manual therapy (use of hands), exercise, hydrotherapy, heat, ultrasound, and electrical stimulation to relieve pain, regain range of movement, and to build strength and flexibility to help improve your health and mobility. Physiotherapists (PTs) have a detailed understanding of how the body works, knowledge of disease, injury and the healing process, and the ability to distinguish what is normal from abnormal in posture, balance, and movement and function.

What Is Physiotherapy Intended to Do?

A good PT encourages you to assume responsibility for your health and participate in a team approach that promotes, restores, and prolongs physical independence. The PT should gather all the necessary information from your health care team and assess which category you are in:

- Osteopenia (mild bone changes) and no fractures but wish to reduce the risk of further bone loss and fractures
- Those with osteoporosis without any fractures
- Those with advanced osteoporosis that have one or more spinal fractures.

He or she should confirm with your doctor if you have primary or secondary osteoporosis. For example, if you have rheumatoid arthritis and have now developed osteoporosis the therapy chosen should be tailored to suit your needs and abilities. The key is for him/her to determine how the disease is affecting you and your lifestyle, which problems are the most important and should be addressed first, what your needs are, and how physiotherapy can reduce or eliminate your problems and enable you to be active again.

Collaboration between your physician and PT can improve your recovery. The physician can provide details on your bone density results and fractures and the PT in turn can share your progress with your physician. If the PT sees that it is unsafe for you to walk independently he/she may advise the physician and determine that you require the use of a walker and assistance from other health professionals to regain mobility (i.e., occupational therapist). If you are continuing to experience intense pain they should advise your physician.

Physiotherapy can help reduce pain, decrease fear of movement, and improve posture and balance. The PT will create a program that is customized to you and fit into your lifestyle so that you are more likely to continue the program on a long-term basis. The goal is to keep you moving! The PT should share information on:

- How to best move to reduce the risk of fractures (i.e., bending and reaching)

- The consequences of immobility

- The risk factors for falling and fall prevention

- The importance of weight bearing activity or resistance activity to strengthen your bones and muscles.

Table 10.1 is a comprehensive list of PT goals for various levels of bone loss (adapted from guidelines endorsed by the Chartered Society of Physiotherapy and the National Osteoporosis Society in the United Kingdom in 2005).

Table 10.1	Osteopenia	Osteoporosis with no fractures	Osteoporosis with one or more fractures
Prevent fractures	√	√	√
Increase BMD	√	√	√
Improve muscle strength, balance, cardiovascular fitness	√	√	√
Improve posture	√	√	√
Build knowledge on osteoporosis	√	√	√
Improve psychological well-being and increase self-confidence	√	√	√
Increase mobility and range of motion		√	√
Improve gait (the way you walk)		√	√
Aim to reduce falls		√	√
How to incorporate exercise into daily life		√	√
Prevent new fractures			√
Decrease and manage pain			√
Improve balance and coordination			√
Maintain or regain independence			√

Individuals with osteoporosis are not required to see a physiotherapist and your doctor may not suggest that you do. Based on how much they helped me regain my ability to perform the tasks that make daily life manageable, I highly recommend that you ask your doctor to refer you to a PT with osteoporosis experience!

What You Can Do

- Ask questions when something is not clear to you or if the information from your PT contradicts your physician
- Be open to making changes in your lifestyle

- Speak up if your pain intensifies after certain exercises or something a physiotherapist has introduced—they can often give you an alternate exercise to strengthen a muscle. Do not suffer in silence!

- Persevere. Take one day at a time and if you are overwhelmed tell the PT

- Ask for feedback and ensure your PT communicates with your doctor on your goals, progress, and results

- Ask your PT for advice on what to do if you have a minor setback or soreness in your back. Your therapist could prescribe stretches that you are able to do at home to relieve stiffness, aches, and pains.

Who Covers the Cost of Physiotherapy?

Funding of physiotherapy services varies across Canada and the US. Generally, in Canada, treatments in a hospital setting are covered by health care plans. Funding varies when offered outside a hospital. Most insurance companies require a referral from your doctor and the license or registration number of the physiotherapist (provided by the regulatory board of the College of Physiotherapy of your province or territory) before reimbursing your costs. Be sure to review your insurance plan and check with your physiotherapist before starting your treatments.

What to Watch For

You can see a PT without a referral from your doctor. However, I recommend that you consult with your physician first so he or she can outline the details of your fracture(s), injuries, and medications which can help the PT.

Physiotherapists can work out of clinics and hospitals and/ or have a private practice. Some will see you in your home. Consult with your doctor, a local osteoporosis support group, or the physiotherapy association in your country (see websites in the Reference & Resource section) to find a reputable physiotherapist.

Tip

After I had fractured my spine, but before I (or my doctors) realized that is what had happened, I did everything imaginable to try and get rid of the pain I felt. I tried physiotherapy at a private clinic that I had used previously for a knee injury. In hindsight this was not a good idea—I did not have a diagnosis and the therapist assumed it was back pain from the caesarian section. I left the treatments in tears and with more pain than when arriving. She insisted that I must work harder at my exercises to regain my strength—including the pelvic tilt which I learned after the fact is more harmful for fractures than good!

My lessons learned from this were:

Listen to your body! I disregarded my pain and my own instincts that were telling me that the treatment from the PT was not working and was actually harmful.

Do not self-diagnose. I went to physiotherapy prior to receiving a diagnosis from a doctor. If you have painful symptoms, see your physician and wait for the results.

Don't second-guess yourself. If you believe the therapist is not qualified or lacks experience seek the services of another therapist. Once I was diagnosed with the fractures, my rheumatologist referred me to a physiotherapist renowned for her work with patients with osteoporosis. At our first appointment, I knew that she was competent and compassionate and I trusted her to help educate and support me in my journey to recovery.

A physiotherapist may use one or more of the following techniques: manual therapy, hydrotherapy, ultrasound, transcutaneous electrical nerve stimulation (TENS), and neuromuscular stimulator (EMS).

Manual Therapy

Manual therapy is a hands-on approach where the PT uses specific techniques with his or her hands to assess and treat a variety of problems and injuries. The goal in manual therapy is to focus on the cause of the problem thereby directly and indirectly treating the symptoms. The skill and experience of the therapist will have an impact on your ability to improve.

Hydrotherapy-the Healing Power of Water
What Is It?

Hydrotherapy is physiotherapy in water. This works well for people who are frail or have fractures, as it can be challenging to begin exercising due to the pain or fear of new injury. Exercise in warm water promotes healing, speeds recovery, and reduces pain, muscle spasms and discomfort.

What Is It Hydrotherapy Intended to Do?

It enables you to begin an exercise program with little resistance. The buoyancy/weightlessness and the warm water allow easier movement with less pain to improve muscle strength and aerobic capacity. And it can make us feel better. The warm water is soothing but also helps boost circulation, release tight muscles, and relieve pain.

The benefits of "water healing" or hydrotherapy have been recognized by many cultures for many years. Think of all the spas that promote healing through water therapies. With a competent physiotherapist and the right guidance and supervision, it can be one of the safest methods for treating people with osteoporotic fractures—especially those suffering from pain and/or postural and balance problems. After the initial fractures there may be exercise that you are unable to do on dry land but are possible in the water.

Fractures can be painful and lead to fear of future fractures. Hydrotherapy allows you to not only build up muscle strength but also the confidence to take on daily activities. People who have a number of problems can feel overwhelmed with fear and the fatigue of long-term pain. The thought of physiotherapy can be daunting. It is also challenging for a physiotherapist to treat everything at once. For people with multiple injuries, hydrotherapy can be a gentle first step to recovery. You can work at balance, strength, flexibility, and pain relief all at the same time with some simple movements in the water. Physiotherapists take their skills and apply them to the water.

They have different philosophies and tricks to help each patient.

What to Watch for

- Be cautious and get assistance getting in and out of the water

- Decide if it is right for you. People with a fear of water will not be relaxed—it may increase anxiety and pain

- Check with your doctor. Hydrotherapy may not be appropriate for people with diabetes or multiple sclerosis and it is not recommended for people with a heart condition, high blood pressure, cardiovascular problems, or a circulation disorder.

> Hydrotherapy proved to be extremely beneficial to me. My mind and body were resistant to engaging in exercises after my fractures. It was just too painful and I did not have the motivation and confidence to begin. When I first submerged my limbs into the over-sized tub I was finally able to relax somewhat and welcome the exercise program. I was able to stand with the support of side bars. I was finally able to do something that would help heal my injuries. It was both soothing and confidence building. It was my first sign that I was going to get better!

Ultrasound

Ultrasound equipment generates low or high frequency sound waves that are transferred to a specific area of your skin via a round-headed wand or probe. The sound waves penetrate the muscles and travels deep into tissue creating gentle heat. Ultrasound gel is used on the surfaces of the body in order to reduce friction and assist in the transmission of the ultrasonic waves. Using gentle, circular motions with the probe, the therapist administers the treatment, which lasts several minutes.

The sound waves that pass through the skin cause a vibration of the local tissues (which feels like a tingling sensation). This vibration can cause a deep heating locally, though usually you won't feel any sensation of heat. Ultrasound can help relax the muscles before or after other treatments, reduce muscle tension and spasms, relieve pain, increase circulation to the area that assists in healing, increase range of motion, and warm muscles before stretching and exercising.

What to Watch for

- Ultrasound demands little from you; however, the results including pain relief produced by ultrasound may only be temporary. It is more effective when used to complement other treatments

- It should not be used for acute inflammation as it may exacerbate the inflammation

- It is for short-term use and normally discontinued once a patient starts to regain strength and begins an exercise program at home

- It should not be used if you have metal implants below the area being treated, you have a local acute infection, or if you have vascular abnormalities (such as blood vessels in poor condition or thrombophlebitis).

Transcutaneous Electrical Nerve Stimulation (TENS)

Transcutaneous (through the skin) electrical nerve stimulation sends a painless electrical current to specific nerves. The mild electrical current generates heat that can relieve stiffness, improve mobility, and relieve acute or chronic pain. Low level electrical current is believed to stimulate the release of endorphins and block pain messages to the brain. The patient wears a small battery-powered device with surface electrodes near the area of pain to provide continuous or intermittent electrical impulses to nerve endings beneath the skin.

The success of TENS depends on many factors, including such things as how long you have had pain, previous treatments, and complementary treatments. Studies on TENS show it is not effective for everyone but some people benefit from its use.

When TENS is used for pain control, a physiotherapist should help you try different frequencies and intensities to find those that provide the best pain control for you. The optimal settings are often determined by trial and error. Also, electrode positioning is quite important. Usually, the electrodes are placed initially on the skin over the painful area, but sometimes moving to other locations (also through trial and error) near the site of pain may give comparable or even better pain relief.

The advantage of TENS is that the stimulator is portable so it can be worn around the waist. The unit can be turned on or off as needed for pain control. Although these units can be purchased or rented, a prescription from a physician is required. The physiotherapist should teach you how to use the device at home.

What to Watch for

- Consult with your doctor prior to using TENS

- TENS should not be used by people with a pacemaker

- A TENS should be used cautiously so be sure to get clear instructions from your PT

- Check with your insurer before using TENS to see whether it is covered for your condition and, if so, to what extent.

Neuromuscular Stimulator

A Neuromuscular stimulator, like a TENS, is a small battery-powered device with electrodes that are affixed to your skin. Neuromuscular stimulation or electronic muscle stimulation (EMS) sends small electrical impulses through the skin to the nerves and muscles to create an involuntary muscle contraction.

EMS is used to re-educate your muscles and increase blood supply to a specific area. When suffering from spinal fractures it is often difficult to begin the necessary exercises to strengthen the muscles to support your back. And when not in use your muscles lose their strength (atrophy). They sometimes need encouragement or re-education to begin working again. The EMS creates involuntary muscle contractions, helping to improve and maintain muscle tone and strength with minimal physical activity.

EMS is still considered experimental and investigational. However, it is commonly used despite the lack of hard scientific evidence to support it.

What to Watch for

- EMS should not be used by some people with severe scoliosis or severe osteoporosis

- The long-term effects of chronic electrical stimulation are unknown

- EMS should not be used by patients with a pacemaker or diagnosed heart problems

- Check with your insurer before using EMS to see whether it is covered for your condition and, if so, to what extent.

Under the guidance of my physiotherapist, I rented and used EMS at home for specific exercises for a few months to reeducate my muscles. I had lost a great deal of muscle after being on bed rest for eight weeks and then suffering from the fractures. At one point I went to do an exercise under the guidance of my physiotherapist and one of my leg muscles just did not respond! I was shocked. I had to truly concentrate on making the muscle work and used EMS to get it "firing" again. Once I gained strength, I graduated to exercises without the EMS.

Osteopathy

Osteopathic Manual Practitioners (OMPs) believe you are more than just the sum of your parts and practice a "whole person" approach to health. Instead of just treating specific symptoms or illnesses, they regard your body as an integrated whole. In short, it means each part of the body affects each and every other part. OMPs have a highly trained sense of touch. The tools OMPs use are their hands. They spend most of their working day with their hands on people—literally feeling what the cause of the problem is, what's not working normally, and working to improve the movement and health in the joints and soft tissue. Treatment is focused on the cause (where possible) rather than just treating the symptoms.

I would say that the difference between a PT and an OMP is the extent to which they look at the impact of the injury on your entire body. Physiotherapists direct their attention to the area where the spinal fractures are and the tissue and muscles surrounding the fractures. An OMP will look further to see how the injury may be affecting other areas of your body. OMPs have a great deal of training in the musculoskeletal system (the interconnected system of nerves, muscles, and bones that make up two-thirds of your body mass). This training provides them with a better understanding of the ways that an injury or illness on one part of your body can affect another. The osteopathic philosophy embraces the notion that the body is naturally able to heal itself.

Osteopathy means that the focus is on the individual person rather than the disease itself. This is very helpful for people with spinal fractures as each individual may be affected somewhat differently by a spinal fracture. The location and impact of pain can vary.

The consultation with the OMP should be a pleasant and relaxing experience. The OMP will use his or her hands to diagnose, treat, and prevent causes of pain, illness or injury. He/she will move your muscles and joints using techniques including stretching, gentle pressure, and resistance.

A typical first visit to the OMP should include the following steps:

1. An interview to learn about your past and present health, including your medical history, problems that are bothering you, any medical treatments, and medications taken, details of the pain you may be experiencing (how strong, when it started, etc.) and your general health.

2. A physical exam to ensure it is safe for you to receive osteopathy treatment. He or she will check your posture, gait, spine, balance, and flexibility. The OMP checks your joints, muscles, tendons, and ligaments and determines where there are any restrictions and how the body is affected by the trauma of the fractures and how the body is adjusting or compensating to these effects.

3. A diagnosis based on the interview and physical exam and what areas of the body are affected by the spinal fractures.

4. A treatment plan to help reduce pain, improve circulation, reduce muscle spasm, improve and maintain flexibility,

maintain nerve supply, restore muscle and joint function, and allow you to become more mobile.

The number of appointments required will be based on you and your body's response to treatment. A good OMP will re-assess you at each appointment as everyone responds differently to therapy. He/she will also give you some good stretching and strengthening exercises to do as homework along with tips on injury prevention. It is important to give feedback to the OMP during the session or after your session if the pain increases and you are uncomfortable.

According to the Canadian College of Osteopathy, there are two groups of professionals who practice osteopathy in Canada:

- Osteopathic physicians are licensed M.D.s who have studied osteopathic manual training at a college approved by the American Osteopathic Association (there are no training centers for osteopathic doctors in Canada). Osteopathic physician in the US must graduate from one of the nation's osteopathic medical schools. Each school is accredited by the American Osteopathic Association's Commission on Osteopathic College Accreditation

- Osteopathic Manual Practitioners (OMPs) have extensive training in manual osteopathic practice, but they are not medical doctors. They treat patients using manual techniques only. The training needed to obtain a diploma in Osteopathic Manual Practice is available in Canada. The program is usually five years of rigorous part-time study followed by a research thesis.

What to Watch for

At the time this book went to print, there were no government regulations for the manual practice of osteopathy in Canada. Some provinces are working on submissions to the provincial governments to ask the government to create regulations for osteopathy. As a result, it is best to do your homework, talk to your health care team, an osteoporosis support group, or check the osteopath associations in your province, state or country for a referral to a reputable OMP who is knowledgeable about osteoporosis and has treated women with spinal fractures.

Both physiotherapy and osteopathy should not be thought of as an alternative to conventional medical treatment. Instead it is complementary to it. PTs and OMPs frequently rely upon the medical profession's diagnostic tools and skills to determine the appropriateness of their treatment.

> I am fortunate as my physiotherapist is also a certified osteo-pathic manual practitioner. She is absolutely amazing! She is knowledgeable, skilled, and supportive. She taught me to listen to my body and see how the fractures were affecting other parts of my body. As an example, spinal fractures can lead to poor posture which causes compression of internal organs which can lead to other ailments such as heartburn. This has at times had an impact on my quality of life.
>
> A physiotherapist may just treat the injury and not discuss or question the impact on the rest of your body. You may have an injury on your lower spine but you may feel pain in your neck or elsewhere in another area of body as the body is trying to realign itself and compensate for the injury which puts stress on other areas. I continue to see my PT regularly for a "tune-up" and when I have recurrent pain or injure my back. She is a critical member of my heath care team.

Occupational Therapy

Stable, able, and strong is the motto of Canada's Occupational Resource site. Occupational therapy is a rehabilitation specialty that is provided by a licensed individual. The occupational therapist (OT) works with people with temporary or permanent disabilities. The primary goal of OT is to enable people to participate in the activities which give meaning and purpose to their lives. It helps people maximize their independence and return to ordinary tasks around home and at work by maximizing physical potential through lifestyle adaptations and possible use of adaptive and assistive tools. The OT will prescribe activities to promote recovery and rehabilitation. Their goal is to help clients have independent, productive, and satisfying lives.

Occupational therapy helps to solve the problems that interfere with your ability to do the things that are important to you. It can also prevent a problem or minimize its effects. When a fracture limits your ability to take care of yourself, participate in paid or unpaid work, or enjoy your leisure time, then an OT can help you learn some new skills for the job of living. Occupational therapists believe that occupations (activities) describe who you are and how you feel about yourself. If you are unable to perform the activities that enable you to live and enjoy your life, your general well-being may be affected.

Occupational therapy can help people resume daily living. The profession takes a broad view of occupation to mean everything people do to participate in daily life. OTs are concerned with developing skills, restoring function and independence, maintaining ability and promoting health and safety to enable individuals to achieve personal goals and occupational performance in the areas of self-care, productivity, and leisure.

Services typically include:

- Customized treatment programs to improve your ability to perform daily activities

- Comprehensive home and job site evaluations with adaptation recommendations

- Performance skills assessments and treatment

- Adaptive equipment recommendations and usage training

- Assessment and management of personal and environmental risk factors

- Training and tips for injury prevention.

Depending on your situation, an OT may check:

- What you can and cannot do physically (this includes your strength, coordination, balance, or other physical abilities)

- What materials you use to participate in the occupation (for example, work tools, furniture, cooking utensils, clothes, or other materials)

- The social and emotional support available to you in your home, school, work, and community

- The physical setup of your house, school, classroom, work place, community, or other environment.

An OT can help you:

- Learn new ways of doing things (e.g., lifting)
- Do activities to help you improve your abilities, strength, and confidence
- Adapt equipment you use (e.g., bath safety devices)
- Make changes to your environment to prevent injury.

What to Watch for

Consult your doctor or other members of your health care team or check the OT website for your province, state or country to get a referral to a reputable occupational therapist. Some OTs specialize in working with a specific age group or condition such as osteoporosis. All provinces and states regulate the practice of occupational therapy.

Who Covers the Cost of Occupational Therapy?

Insurance coverage and availability of OT services varies across Canada and the US. In Canada, your family doctor can refer you to an OT for services covered under your provincial medical plan. These OTs usually work in hospitals or government-funded rehabilitation centers and home care programs. If you have extended health care benefit insurance, your plan may cover OT services. The Canadian Association of Occupational Therapists and its provincial affiliates are lobbying insurance companies to include occupational therapy as an insured benefit on their plans. Be sure to review your insurance plan and check with your OT before your treatments.

Prior to my spinal fractures I was a highly active and independent woman. Relying on others daily to shower, dress, and pick up any item I dropped on the floor made me angry and humiliated. Yet I was stubborn. I did not readily accept the devices offered to me by the occupational therapist to improve my daily living. I gradually relented and swallowed my pride, which allowed me to lead a more independent life while my fractures were healing. The OT showed me new ways of doing things and suggested many devices. These included:

- A walker

- A shower bar

- A sock-aid

- A railing for the front step

- A "reacher" to help me pick up items that dropped to the floor.

OTs are very valuable as they help people like me lead independent, productive, and satisfying lives.

There are many options to choose from to regain your quality of life. Getting well is a team effort. You need to take an active role in your recovery. A good therapist will promote this and guide you on how to help yourself. After all, the primary goal is to be pain free, strong, and independent as soon as possible! A good therapist gets a lot of pleasure from knowing that you have recovered enough to no longer need his or her services. But knowing and meeting the therapist who is right for you is just the beginning—active exercise and home programs are crucial elements that will help speed your recovery.

CHAPTER 11

~

BETTER BONES
THROUGH EXERCISES

When I began physiotherapy I was very weak, fragile, and in a great deal of pain. I had no desire to get out of bed, let alone exercise. Meeting my physiotherapist gave me the momentum I needed to become active instead of passive in my rehabilitation. Each weekly home physiotherapy session was a building block to strengthen my muscles. I also exercised and stretched daily using a program that she created for me. Although I felt like my progress was moving at a snail's pace, each gain gave me the motivation I needed to keep up my program. My sessions started at home, progressed to weekly treatments with my PT at the hospital with hydrotherapy, and then to monthly visits. Eventually I graduated to using a weekly exercise regime designed by a personal trainer and life wellness coach. Although I have gained muscle and strength, the shape of my spine has been altered forever, so I continue to see my PT for "tune-ups" or when I have an injury that causes pain. I cannot pretend that this process was easy. In fact, it was one of the most difficult periods of my life. Just thinking about it as I wrote this chapter brought back many painful memories. But it is important to know that you can and will regain physical strength and manage this disease.

My top lesson learned from both my PT and trainer is that posture must be a priority. When walking by a mirror I am often shocked to see how my posture dwindles as the day progresses. I think I am standing tall but I am not. Due to fatigue—maybe even laziness—my shoulders are hunched and my head is jutting forward. When I catch a glimpse of this it signals me to realign my spine by following the simple steps in this chapter.

Building better bones and muscles is up to you! For many doctors, the focus is on reviewing your Bone Mineral Density (BMD) and your blood work to evaluate your risk for fracture, then deciding on the optimal medication to improve your bone health. Due to time constraints and not necessarily being their area of expertise, exercise is rarely discussed other than as a question to find out if you exercise. You will need initiative to start and build momentum with an exercise program but I can assure you that this will give you the greatest joy and return on investment of your time. Think of your exercise minutes as dollars in your bone bank and make an investment in your bone health each day.

Why Exercise?

John Hopkins University, a world leader in medical research, reported on the findings of a study from the University of Arizona confirming that the combination of increased physical activity and improved nutrition does help prevent bone loss. Results from the study show that women who followed a regimen of weight-bearing and resistance exercises faithfully for four years, while taking calcium citrate supplements, had significant improvement in BMD at key skeletal sites. There are many studies that provide evidence that even though you have been diagnosed with osteoporosis and have sustained a fracture, you can improve your bone density and muscle strength.

The right exercise and activities will help bring back joy in your life and avoid broken bones. The benefits are enormous! Here is a list of just some of the aims of exercise:

- Improve bone density
- Improve flexibility
- Improve posture and prevent stooped or slumping posture
- Improve balance and coordination and reduce risk of falls
- Release natural endorphins to reduce pain, help your mood, and prevent depression
- Increase your energy level

- Grow confidence.

The role of exercise in enhancing your quality of life cannot be underestimated!

Before You Start an Exercise Program

- **Consult with your doctor before starting any exercises.** Any exercise program can be a risk, especially for someone with osteoporosis. I hesitated to add any exercises in this chapter for fear that readers would begin them without consulting with their physician. However, I want to ensure that readers understand the importance of exercise in managing osteoporosis and maintaining an active lifestyle. Please review the exercises in this chapter with your doctor

- **Consult with an exercise expert**. Do your homework. Ask your doctor or a local osteoporosis support group or others living with osteoporosis for a referral to a reputable professional who has a solid knowledge of osteoporosis. Find the right team member—a health professional to develop and guide you through an exercise program (i.e., a physiotherapist, Osteopathic Manual Practitioner, certified fitness consultant, certified athletic therapist or kinesiologist with expertise in osteoporosis and helping people with fractures)

- **Find a good listener**. If you find the professional inexperienced, incompetent, or not listening to your needs, find another who will!

- **Never curl the spine** and bend forward at the waist—called spinal flexion—because of risk of compression fracture (e.g., sit-ups or bending over to touch your toes)

- **Do not do exercises that twist the spine**

- **Avoid high impact exercises**. Examples include running, some aerobics, skipping, and jumping

- **Set goals**. Write them down and celebrate successes

- **Wear comfortable clothing.** Proper shoes with good support are essential

- **Learn to recognize the difference between discomfort and pain**. Pain is the body's way of telling you something is wrong. Listen to your body. Muscle fatigue is okay. Total body fatigue is not. Do not continue to exercise when you cannot hold correct form. Good body mechanics is the best injury prevention

- **Aim to do your exercises in the morning**. Research shows that those who do this tend to stick with their program.

Tips when Exercising

- Listen to your body! If you have any pain stop the exercise immediately. I can't stress this strongly enough.

- Exercises should be tailored to you and your abilities.

- Exercises should be progressive and enjoyable.

- You are more likely to stick to a program that is convenient, doable, and at a pace that is comfortable for you.

- If you are uncomfortable with an exercise and fear injury, tell your trainer and ask for a different exercise that will help build that muscle.

- Start with 3-5 repetitions and build up gradually to 8-10 repetitions.

- Do the exercises slowly. You get more benefit from an exercise done correctly three times than rushing through eight haphazard repetitions.

- Ensure your expert revises your program periodically to work various muscles.

- Consider seeking out an exercise partner so you can encourage each other to continue each of your exercise regimens.

- Begin at a low level and progress gradually.

Posture

Osteoporosis can be nasty to your posture. This change often involves a stooped posture with the shoulders rounding forward and a forward-bending position from the hips. This posture can lead to chronic back pain and can restrict breathing. Also the shoulder, back, and chest muscles can become tight which often leads to problems with grooming and dressing. Since some of these postural changes are muscular in nature they can be corrected with simple exercises.

You can protect your bones and muscles by practicing proper posture and learning the correct way to move. One of the most important concepts in body mechanics and posture is alignment, which refers to the relationship of the head, shoulders, spine, and hips to one another. Proper alignment puts less stress on the spine and ensures good posture. The average weight of the head is incredibly heavy—between 4.5 and 5.0 kilograms (10 or 11 pounds). A slumped, head-forward posture puts harmful stress on the spine, as does bending forward or twisting your spine.

The key to all exercises and activities is to maintain a neutral spine. A neutral spine is the natural position of the spine when all three curves of the spine—cervical (neck), thoracic (middle), and lumbar (lower)—are present and in good alignment. This is the strongest position for the spine when we are standing or sitting, and the one that we are made to move from as it minimizes stress on the joints, muscles and vertebrae. Not only does it feel good—it looks good, bringing a longer, leaner appearance to your body.

To properly align your spine into a neutral posture:

- Stand with your back against a wall with your heels one inch from the wall

- Tighten your abdominal muscles and flatten your back against the wall. One way to do this is to think of a zipper pulling up your tummy muscles

- Lift your chest, keep your head up and look straight ahead

- Bring your shoulders back toward the wall. There should be a small hollow at the small of your back

- Tuck your chin in and make sure it is not jutting out

- Maintaining this position, move away from the wall and check your posture in a full-length mirror from the front and side. Continue to breath slowly (don't hold your breath)

- Check your posture in a mirror to see if your body is in alignment when exercising and a few times throughout the day

- Practicing and sustaining this posture position regularly can help the body record and store the movement as new muscle memory. As one of my "bone angels," personal trainer Catherine Morisset says, "Be long, stable, and strong!"

Breathing

Breathing properly during exercise can mean the difference between actually completing the exercise or not. It really is that important. Learning how to breathe correctly while you exercise can change your entire experience when exercising. It may sound simplistic but proper breathing is key to getting oxygen to all your muscles, clearing your body of carbon dioxide and preventing your blood pressure from rising, which can cause unpleasant dizziness.

The general rule of thumb when exercising is to exhale on exertion (the hard part of the movement) and inhale during the easier part of a movement. On a push-up against a wall, for example, you inhale on the way down and exhale when you are pushing up away from the wall.

People often unknowingly hold their breath when exercising. We get so caught up in the effort that we forget to breathe! Try to use your normal breathing pattern or do your best to increase the length of your inhales and exhales. Also, if you are having trouble catching your breath—slow down. Take a few minutes to focus on your breathing before you start moving to help set the rhythm for your exercises.

Water

Is water important? Absolutely! Water makes up 75% of your body, regulates body temperature, helps your breathing, transports nutrients, carries away waste, and helps your muscles function. Without water, your muscles become dehydrated. Muscle movement depends on how hydrated you are, so if muscles are dry, they will not work as well. Being dehydrated can sap your energy and make you feel tired. If you're thirsty, you're already dehydrated—and this can slow you down and make it harder to complete your routine. It can also lead to fatigue, muscle weakness, dizziness, and other symptoms.

When we exercise we tend to dry out. During 20 minutes of vigorous exercise, the average person can sweat more than one cup of fluid! As you can see, exercise saps a lot of water from our bodies. That's why it's very important to drink water before, during, and after exercising.

The American College of Sports Medicine (ACSM) points out that as we get older, drinking enough water is especially important because with age our body is less able to regulate our temperature, putting us at increased risk of heat-related illness. Age also affects our ability to stay hydrated during exercise and our ability to recognize when we need more water. Being hydrated is part of your bone building workout. Forming the habit isn't hard, with a little focus.

Tips:
- Start paying attention to your daily fluid intake.
- Before exercising drink one cup of water.
- Keep a water bottle with you and take sips between exercises.
- Drink another cup after you exercise.
- Keep replenishing your fluid levels by drinking water regularly throughout the day.
- Try to generally keep yourself from getting thirsty.
- Don't force yourself to drink large amounts of water.

The more you drink before, during, and after exercise, the more productive your exercise program will be. Do your body a favor and replenish the fluids your body is losing while you work out. Your muscles will thank you later.

Exercises

Choosing the right form of exercise is key. You want to ensure you have a safe, effective, and enjoyable regimen that boosts your bone health and enhances your quality of life after fracture. Three types of activities are recommended for people with osteoporosis:

- Flexibility exercises

- Strength training exercises

- Weight-bearing aerobic activities.

Think about making a one-month commitment to exercise. If you are able to increase your physical activity for 30 days, that's a good sign that you are on your way to making exercise and physical activity regular, life-long habits. I have provided an introductory program of gentle exercises that you can review with your exercise specialist.

Table 11.1

Type of Exercise	Why?	Minimum Time
Warm-up	To warm up muscles, increase blood flow to working muscles and the heart, prevent injury, reduce stiffness and help clear your mind	5 minutes of moderate walking (treadmill or natural) priorto doing any type of exercise
Flexibility Exercises/Stretches	Improves flexibility, relieves tension, helps prevent slumping forward during the day	10 minutes daily
Weight-bearing aerobic	Boosts your heart and circulatory system Slows bone loss Stimulates bone building	20-30 minutes Five times/week
Strength or resistance training	Improves postural stability (balance) Strengthens muscles supporting the spine Prevents falls & improves gait (the way you walk)	Three times per week
Cool-down	Helps reduce stiffness and soreness	Walk slowly for 3-5 (treadmill or natural) minutes and breathe slowly & deeply

Important—If you have (or are at risk for) fractures, you MUST consult with your physician before trying ANY exercise. The risk of new injury is simply too great.

Flexibility Exercises/Stretches

Our bodies are not designed to stay in one position all day long, but after spinal fracture(s) you may find yourself instinctively staying in one or two protective positions. Taking regular stretch breaks throughout the day to stretch our major muscle groups can help reduce injury and stiffness. Stretching improves flexibility, helps maintain good balance, prevents muscle injury, and improves posture. Stretches are best performed when your muscles are warmed up. They can be done after aerobic exercises or strengthening exercises. They can also be done periodically throughout the day, especially if you are sitting at a computer for an extended period of time. They should be done gently and slowly, without bouncing.

The key to stretching is to relax and focus on the area being stretched. Stretches should feel good and not be painful. Avoid stretches that twist or flex your spine or cause you to bend at the waist, such as touching your toes. These positions put excessive stress on the vertebrae in your spine, placing you at greater risk of a compression fracture. To help guide you, the References & Resources section provides websites with videos and illustrations of the following stretches and exercises.

Seven Stretches to Help Stand Tall

Gentle Neck stretch

Stand (with feet hip-width apart) or sit with a neutral posture. Relax your shoulders and have your arms hanging loosely at sides. Look straight forward. Place your index finger on your chin and give it a gentle push to ensure it is tucked in and that your head is aligned with your spine and not jutting out. Slowly tilt your left ear to your left shoulder until you feel a gentle stretch on the right side of your neck. Do not bounce. Don't bring your shoulder up to your ear. Hold for 10-20 seconds and relax. Repeat five times on each side.

Shoulder shrug

To loosen your shoulders and neck, shrug your shoulders up slowly toward your ears (avoid jerky movements) while holding your arms at your sides. Hold for five seconds and then relax your shoulders downward into your normal position. Repeat five times.

Back stretches (these can be done on a floor or firm bed)
Straight leg raise-hamstring stretch

Lie flat on your back, bend both knees. Support the left thigh by placing your hands behind the knee. Slowly attempt to straighten the left leg as much as possible while maintaining a comfortable stretch in the thigh and keeping the back firmly on the bed or floor. Relax and breathe. Hold for a count of 20. Lower your leg slowly. Repeat five times for both legs.

Low back stretch

Lie flat on your back. Bend both knees. Relax, pull tummy muscles in and then using your hands slowly pull your left leg toward your chest until a comfortable stretch is felt in your back. Keep the back of your head on the floor. Do not strain. Hold for 20 seconds. Repeat five times for both legs.

Standing stretch

Standing with spine in neutral position, interlace your fingers behind your back. Slowly turn your elbows inward while straightening your arms. Hold for 10 seconds. Repeat three times.

Leg stretch

While sitting with a neutral posture, keep the balls of your feet on the floor and raise your heels. Hold for 10 seconds. Lower your heels back down, and repeat 10 times. Although this is really a calf stretch exercise, you'll feel the stretch all the way up into your lower back.

Calf stretch

Stand approximately 60-90 centimeters (two to three feet) facing a bare wall. Make certain there is nothing on the ground between you and the wall. Start with a neutral posture. Place your hands shoulder width apart against the wall with your palms flat and elbows slightly bent. Take one step forward with your left foot, toes pointing forward and heel on the ground. Bend your left knee slowly, using the movement to control the amount of stretch you feel in your right calf muscle. Both heels stay on the ground. Keep your right knee (back leg) straight and hold stretch for 10 seconds. Do not bounce. Move gently and slowly to return back to the starting position. Repeat three times with each leg.

Weight-bearing Aerobic Activities

Weight-bearing aerobic activities (bones and muscles work against the force of gravity) are the most beneficial in stimulating bone-building. They involve aerobic exercise on your feet, with your bones supporting your weight. A weight-bearing exercise does not need to be a high-impact exercise like jogging. Examples include walking on your own or on a treadmill machine, Nordic walking (walking with poles), and stair climbing. These types of exercises work directly on the bones in your legs, hips, and lower spine to slow mineral loss. The key is to choose exercises that boost the heart and bones at the same time. Aim to walk at a moderate or brisk pace for at least five minutes and build up to 20 minutes. If winter poses a problem because of icy conditions or if you are not able to walk comfortably unaided, try a treadmill that you can hold on to and begin at a very low speed and incline and gradually build up your time and slope degree.

Water Exercises

If you are not yet able to walk without pain, then water or aqua aerobics in a pool may be your exercise of choice. They are designed to improve cardiovascular function, strengthen and condition muscles, and decrease back pain. The water's buoyancy reduces injury risk as the joints are exposed to less stress and impact. Exercising in water helps increase the endurance and strength of muscles but cannot increase low bone density. It can help build your confidence and be a stepping stone to exercises outside of the pool.

Some pools have lifts, if stairs in and out of the pool are an issue. You can also find water shoes with "sticky" grips designed for pool side walking (these can be worn into the pool, if you wish). If you are comfortable in the water, you may find the zero impact of a deep water workout even more appealing—water wings will add both resistance and safety.

Strength Training

Strength training—also called resistance training—uses various means of resistance such as free weights, weight machines, resistance bands, and water exercises to strengthen the muscles and bones in your arms and upper spine. It can also work directly on your bones to slow mineral loss. The force your muscles exert on the bones helps to strengthen them. The stronger a muscle is, the more force it exerts upon the bone. Therefore, by strengthening your muscles you can also strengthen your bones.

Resistance exercises move objects or your own body weight to create resistance. As they contract against the resistance (water, dumbbells, rubber tubing) muscle mass builds and bones associated with the muscle group strengthen through an osteogenic, or bone-building, effect. Trabecular bone responds best to this type of exercise. If your recall from Chapter 5, bones in the spine and hip are predominantly trabecular bone.

It is essential to find an exercise professional with experience in osteoporosis to design a strength-training program that is appropriate for your fractures and degree of bone loss and to teach you the proper techniques to avoid injury. My trainer strongly urges her clients to use resistance bands over weights as they benefit more muscles and reduce the chance of injury.

The Importance of a Strong Core

"Core" is a word that is used frequently by exercise specialists. When we talk about the core we are grouping the muscles that make a strong connection between our lower and upper body, the "core." Having a strong core will make our bodies more resilient to the external forces that are applied to our bodies daily. Even opening a door requires some core strength, otherwise as our hand meets with the door our upper body will collapse. Core exercises train the muscles in the pelvis, lower back, hips, and abdomen to work in harmony. This leads to better balance and stability in daily activities. Most sports and other physical activities depend on stable core muscles.

In general the core muscles run the length of the trunk and torso. When they contract they stabilize the spine, pelvis, and shoulders and create a solid base of support. It pays to get your core muscles—

the muscles around your trunk and pelvis—in better shape. Core exercises strengthen your abdominal muscles, pelvis, and mid and lower back, making most physical activities easier. Focus on tightening your deepest abdominal muscle—the transversus abdominis—during each exercise. This is the muscle you feel contracting when you cough.

Research indicates that strengthening your back muscles helps treat osteoporosis by maintaining or improving posture. That's because the stooped posture caused by osteoporotic compression fractures may cause increased pressure along your spine, leading to even more compression fractures. Exercises that gently arch your back can strengthen back muscles while minimizing stress on bones.

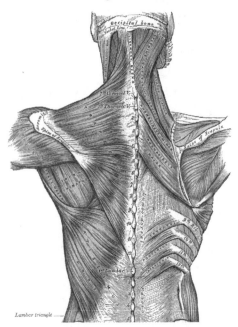

Figure 11.1 Muscles Supporting The Spine

Because many of the more common core strengthening exercises involve spinal compression and twisting (e.g., sit-ups), it is important that your core program is designed by a trainer who understands osteoporosis and potential dangers to the spine.

Working on Bones & Muscles & Building Your Core

Wall push-ups

Stand approximately 60-90 centimeters (two to three feet) facing a bare wall. Make certain there is nothing on the ground between you and the wall. Start with a neutral posture. Place your hands shoulder width apart against the wall with your palms flat. Your arms should be straight, but avoid locking your elbows when in the starting position. While keeping your heels on the floor and body in a straight line (maintaining that neutral posture, tummy tuck) do push-ups against the wall by leaning in until your nose is approximately five centimeters (two inches from the wall). Keep your eyes focused straight ahead and only bend as far as comfortable. Slowly push out with your arms to return to your starting position. Repeat 5-10 times or until it becomes challenging to return to the starting position.

Wall arm raises or wall arm presses

Stand and face a wall with your nose touching the wall. Start with a neutral posture-tummy and chin tucked in. Place your arms against the wall at shoulder level, palms facing the wall. As you inhale, slowly slide your extended arms up the wall with your thumbs leading the way. Only go as a far as you can while keeping a neutral posture. Repeat 5-10 times.

Sitting knee extension to strengthen thighs

Sit in a chair with your back and hips against the back of the chair and your feet flat against the floor. Start with a neutral posture—tummy and chin tucked in. Place your hands on your thighs and look straight ahead. Slowly straighten the left knee while lifting your heel a few inches from the floor. Only go as far as you can while maintaining a good posture. Don't slouch or round your back. Hold this position for a count of 10 while breathing normally. Relax and return to the starting position. Repeat 5-10 times with each leg.

Calf raises

Stand about 30 centimetres (about one foot) behind the back of a chair with feet hip-width apart and knees slightly bent. Keep back in a neutral position, head in line with spine, and shoulders back. Use the chair for balance and do not lean forward. Slowly raise heels off the floor, pushing straight up onto balls of your feet. Pause one second, then slowly lower heels to starting position. Complete 5-10 repetitions.

Leg extensions

Stand up straight in a neutral position with head in line with spine, legs hip-width apart and knees straight. Place your hands on the back of a chair for balance. Maintaining good posture, breathe, and slowly raise your left leg upwards by lifting your foot 10 centimeters off the floor (a few inches). Keep a good posture and be sure not to lean forward. Pause for one second. Lower left leg to the floor. Complete 5 to 10 repetitions with each leg.

Mid-back exercise with resistance band

Stand with your back to a wall with knees soft and feet shoulder-width apart. Check to ensure you have a neutral posture with tummy and chin tucked in. Seeing yourself in a mirror can help. Grasp the resistance band with your hands, arms straight with hands at waist level. With your palms facing the floor, slowly pull arms away from each other, ending with your arms open and touching the wall. Maintain good posture with eyes forward and band no higher than your lower ribs. Count to three and release gently and slowly to starting position. Repeat five times.

Exercise is a critical step to building better bones and managing and even overcoming pain. The key is to consult with your doctor and an exercise expert, set realistic goals, take baby steps, and celebrate successes. The rewards are incredible:

- It rebuilds strength that is often lost following a spinal fracture, due to restricted movement

- It gave me the confidence to go about my daily activities with much less fear of injury

- It mitigated the osteoporosis spinal "slump" so that I look and feel better.

In darker moments, my osteoporosis and spinal fractures diagnosis made me feel powerless. But seeing my strength and capacity increase as I continued to exercise made me feel powerful. It renewed my hope that I would be able to get my life back. Since I achieved that goal, I find that regular exercise helps both my bone health and my attitude!

Now let's look at simple strategies to keep your bones and body happy throughout the day.

CHAPTER 12

~

STAND STRONG AFTER SPINAL FRACTURE

Body Mechanics & Posture

You can protect your bones by practicing proper posture and learning the correct way to move (called body mechanics). Correct body movements can reduce pain and reduce risk of injury after fracture. When you move your body in your everyday activities, you want to move in a way that promotes healing and prevents injury. Bad body mechanics are bad for the bones! They can result in injuries to the vertebrae, discs, and back muscles—and can cause the back to become less stable.

After standing tall and strong by properly aligning the spine and checking your posture from the front and side in the mirror (as outlined in Chapter 11), there are minor adjustments you can make to your body to prevent injury while you are active throughout the day. While you may think that this is common sense, many people, including myself, have suffered the consequences of practicing poor body mechanics. We bend, lift, reach, and twist without proper body mechanics, especially when in a hurry. For me it often happens when I am dashing out the door with my nine-year-old daughter. Something as simple as bending and lifting winter boots out of a hallway closet has cost me dearly. I may not feel any stress on my back at the time, but the activities that I regained through massive effort can come screeching to a halt the next day. I then face two to three weeks of gut wrenching pain and a few trips to physiotherapy before I experience relief.

Here are some tips I have gathered to help you move safely while standing, sitting, walking, bending, lifting, gardening, and performing other regular daily activities along with information on sports that are hard on the spine and travel tips (because I love traveling and felt it was a huge victory when I was able to take my first post-fracture trip).

Before any Activities

When you begin your day, check to see that you have a neutral spine and focus briefly on your abdominal, hip, and back muscles. These are the muscles that hold your back in the neutral position. It may seem like golf at first, where you have to consciously plot out the steps before you take that swing–but soon the steps become natural habits that are part of your day-to-day life. Scientists say that it takes 21 days to create a new habit. You can start today!

When Standing

- Wear shoes that provide support both for the back and for the arches of your feet

- Keep your head high, tuck your chin in, and shoulder blades slightly "pinched" together

- Maintain the natural arch of your lower back as you gently pull in your stomach (think of a zipper pulling in your tummy)

- Point your feet straight ahead with your knees facing forward and behind toes

- If you are standing in one place for any length of time, (such as the kitchen) especially on a hard surface, put one foot up on a stool or in an open low cupboard. Switch feet periodically. This will be less tiring for your back and legs.

When Sitting

- When sitting, the entire body weight transfers to your bottom and to your thighs and at the same time it stresses your back and neck to a great extent. Sitting for hours can cause excessive pressure on inter-vertebral discs (the shock absorbing parts of your spinal cord) and blood flow to the heart becomes sluggish

- Sit down slowly and don't plop yourself into a chair as it may jar your back (I have done this). Use a small pillow to support your lower back. The support should be thick enough to cushion your lower back and maintain the normal arch. You should have a natural inward curve to your lower back and a tall, upright upper back

- Look straight ahead, keep back and hips in alignment, and your hips and knees at the same level. If your feet do not rest flat on the floor, use a small footstool

- When using the computer keep your ears lined with the tops of your shoulders, and shoulders in line with your hips. Push your hips as far back as they can go in the chair and feet flat on the floor or try placing a wedge-shaped block or angled footrest under your feet to tilt your toes slightly upwards. This helps reduce the strain on your back. Position the keyboard so that it is directly in front of you and place the monitor about one arm's length (20 to 26 inches) away. Stand up and stretch frequently using stretches from Chapter 11

- Limit use of your laptop on your lap. Try to use it at a desk and use an external mouse. Your arms and shoulders will be less tense. Linking and using an external keyboard is even better. This means that you can raise your laptop screen to the right level (your head should be slightly inclined down) and type comfortably. Your eyes should roughly be at the same level as the top of the screen. Some laptops have height adjustments for their screens

- When putting on socks or shoes or drying your feet after a shower, sit in a chair and bring your foot up to you, keeping a neutral spine or place one foot on a footstool, box, or on your other leg. Lean forward at the hips to tie or dry. Do not bend over or slouch through your upper back. Keep the natural curve of your lower back and a straight upper back. This is one activity I find challenging and have to be very conscious of doing this correctly. Giving myself a toe treatment is now out of the question, so instead of dwelling on what I can't do, I treat myself to a pedicure!

- Use a footstool or footrest when seated for long periods of time

- When sitting in bucket seats or soft couches or chairs, use a small pillow to support your lower back or an Obus Forme back support

- When reading, do not lean over your work, but maintain a neutral spine. Set your reading material on a pillow on your lap

- When getting out of a chair, scoot your hips to the front of the chair, feet straight ahead, lean your torso forward a bit from the hips and use your leg, hip, and gluteus maximus (buttocks!) muscles to lift yourself up.

When Walking

- Walk tall and strong with a neutral spine

- Wear flat, sturdy, comfortable shoes with good support

- Keep your head held high, chin tucked in, chest up, shoulders relaxed and shoulder blades slightly "pinched"

- Keep your eyes focused on where you are going in lieu of tilting your head down and looking down at your feet on the ground. Point your feet straight ahead, not out to one side, and be sure your toes are not curled

- When you walk, step from heel to toe. Start slowly at a comfortable pace. Build up to a moderate pace

- Do not let your knees lock back as you bring your weight over your foot, but keep them slightly bent. Swing your arms

- Keep hips, knees, and toes properly lined up when climbing stairs

- Be cautious when walking outdoors. Avoid jolting the spine when stepping off a curb. I have jolted my spine a number of times when I didn't notice changes in pavement levels and it is extremely painful.

When Bending & Lifting

- A neutral spine and bent knees are key. Even light items require careful attention.

- Stand with your feet flat, about shoulder width apart from one another, and one foot slightly ahead of the other. Bend your knees and hips and maintain a neutral spine

- Test the weight of the load first and get help if it is heavy or bulky. Hug the load. Bring the item close to your body at waist level. Gently breathe in and lift by using your leg, thigh, and buttock muscles (not your lower back muscles) to do the bulk of the work to lift the object and straighten up. When you reach an upright position, exhale

- If turning, don't twist. Turn your feet by taking small steps. If carrying is necessary, be sure to pull in your tummy and maintain a neutral spine

- With overhead reaching, use a safe stool to bring yourself up to the level of the object and get as close as possible

- To lower the load, again maintain a neutral spine and squat with your knees and hips.

Tips When Bending & Lifting

- Don't carry heavy objects (such as purses or backpacks) on one side of your body.

- Keep frequently used items in places where you do not have to stretch to reach them. My kitchen was redesigned to avoid having to reach and twist to get items. Many lower shelves were removed and replaced with practical drawers that slide out easily.

- Store heavy items at waist height and lighter items on higher and lower shelves. This will prevent the need to lift heavy items overhead which can cause excessive stress to your back.

- Push versus pull an item if possible. Pushing uses the strong muscles of the legs and hips, while pulling tends to use the muscles of the back. Use your weight to push, lean into the item, bending at the hips and knees and keeping your back straight.

- Don't jerk the object. Lift and move slowly, smoothly, and carefully. Once the object is in motion, follow through as starting and stopping the movement is more difficult and causes more stress to the back.

- When carrying groceries, ask that the bags be packed light! Divide heavy items into separate bags and hold bags close to your body. You may also use a cart with wheels to transport bags from the store to home or from the car into the house. When unpacking, place packages on a chair or counter top instead of the floor.

Proper posture and good body mechanics are important for everyone, especially those with osteoporosis. Think before you lift! When my daughter was only four-months-old, my endocrinologist advised me not to lift my daughter for one year as the risk of another fracture was so high. The most natural activity in the world, picking up my child, was dangerous to me. Many of the activities in this chapter seem so simple to most people, yet for someone with spinal factures the simple act of putting on nylons and shoes can be a challenge.

Bathing

Warm water can soothe the spirit as well as feel like a massage on the muscles, but make sure you practice bathing safety:

- While standing in the shower, maintain a neutral posture and use a long-handled bath sponge to wash yourself below the knees

- In the tub, avoid sitting with your legs straight. Instead, bend one knee to help support your back. Before you sit down in the tub or get out of it, go to a kneeling position and keep your back in the neutral position

- Invest in grab bars for the shower and tub. There is a wide range of equipment available (from simple to sophisticated items) which can help overcome this difficulty. The combination of a seat, grab rails and a slip resistant mat may satisfy your needs.

Because of changes to the shape of my spine I am no longer very comfortable in a tub so I prefer to stick to showers.

Standing at the Bathroom Sink

While brushing your teeth, put one hand on the sink to help support your weight or place one foot on a low stool to help take pressure off your back. When you need to lean over, keep your back in the neutral position and bend at the hips and knees to lower yourself to the level of the sink. Do not slump over or lean uncomfortably far forward. Guilty! This is one activity that I really have to ensure I am doing correctly.

Chores & Household Activities

For the person with osteoporosis, proper body mechanics are essential when performing chores such as vacuuming, mopping, sweeping, and raking.

- To avoid fatigue, try to break these duties up into smaller time periods. I am so guilty of doing too much! If your back and body are sending you signals that fatigue is setting in, such as twinges, stop, take a rest break, and continue later or the next day

- Always face your work directly to keep from twisting your back. Keep your feet apart with one foot in front of the other. Shift your weight from one leg to the other to move the vacuum, broom, mop, or rake back and forth

- Lean forward from the hips, keep your back in a neutral position and bend at the knees instead of the waist. Avoid polishing floors to a high gloss, which makes them slippery. If you wish to scrub a spot on the floor on your hands and knees, that's fine as long as you can move up and down from the floor

- Use the arms and leg muscles while keeping the back in a neutral position. Avoid twisting movements. Use body weight to help with the job

- Get rid of the Martha Stewart syndrome where your home must be perfect—there are some days where the fatigue may be so overwhelming that tidying up and cleaning is impossible. If you can, delegate to someone in the family or, if feasible, hire someone who can do it for you

- Always keep the device (i.e., rake or mop) as directly in front of you as possible. Don't stretch forward while doing theses chores

- If making beds do so from a chair or kneeling or squatting position. Do not lean forward and curve your spine

- Gardening and yard work require long periods of bending forward. Interrupt these activities frequently.

When Getting In or Out of Bed

Be sure to follow the simple and safe steps to get in and out of bed outlined in Chapter 7, *Bedrest & the Road to Recovery*.

When Getting In & Out of a Car

To get into a car, open the door completely and stand with your back to the door opening, facing away from the car. Place one hand on the back of the car seat and one on the dashboard or steering wheel for support as you gently sit down on the car seat leaving both feet outside the vehicle. Using your hands for support on the dashboard, steering wheel, or car seat, turn and rotate your body as one unit to bring yourself into a forward facing position with both legs in the car.

To get out of the car safely, first open the door completely, then swing your legs out to the side and pivot on your buttocks so your entire body moves as a unit. Do not twist the lower back. Place one hand on the seat and the other hand on the car frame. Scoot forward and place feet under the hips, lean forward, and push with one hand while pulling with the other hand. Use the leg muscles to come up to a standing position.

When Reaching

Use both arms together to avoid twisting your spine. Don't reach for a shelf higher than you can easily reach with both arms. Stand on a safety step stool with high handrails or use a reaching device, but lift only lightweight objects. Reorganize work areas so items that are used regularly are stored at waist or eye level.

Bless You! When Coughing or Sneezing

A simple sneeze can travel over 100 mph. With that kind of rocket propulsion force, injuries can happen. Sneezing can aggravate previous back injuries. In rare cases the trauma can cause a spinal fracture. When you sneeze violently and the force throws your body out of kilter it is called whiplash—your head moves forwards and backwards very quickly—and can cause all sorts of damage to muscles, joints, discs, or even vertebrae.

If you want to sneeze safely, you have to brace yourself for the onslaught. Engage your abdominal muscles—remember to "zip" in your tummy—when you feel a sneeze or cough coming. Develop the habit of supporting your back with one hand. This protects the spine, muscles, and disks from damage caused by a sudden bend forward. Never suppress a sneeze, as that can wreak serious injury in the eardrum, blood vessels, or sinus cavities in the head.

During the early stages of my recovery from the fractures, I had a sneeze and ooooooooooh… agony shot through me! It set me back a few weeks. I was dumbfounded that something so common could cause such pain.

Gardening

Gardening can be tough on your back, but for many people gardening is a passion. Good news—gardening, done safely, can be good for the bones! In 2002, University of Arkansas scientists found that strenuous yard work (pulling weeds) had the same beneficial effect on bone density as weight training did. And being among plants and flowers in the sunshine can boost your vitamin D and brings emotional benefits. These simple tips can keep gardening from becoming a backbreaking chore:

* Take a few minutes to stretch before you begin digging or weeding

* Keep a neutral spine

* Have someone load and unload bags of dirt and any other heavy items

* Remember to use proper body mechanics previously described in this chapter when lifting and carrying items—no bending and twisting

- Use raised flower beds that require less bending and stooping
- When doing tasks at ground level, like weeding or planting, kneel rather than bend from the waist. Where possible, keep one hand on the ground for support as you lean forward
- Step into the flower bed to work rather than lean in from the edge
- Aim to work on "all fours" maintaining a normal spinal curvature and supporting some of your weight with your arms. Use foam pads to protect your knees when on the hard ground
- Use long-handled tools with good grip surface
- Take frequent breaks to stop, rest, and "smell the roses!"
- Listen to your body. If it hurts stop and take a rest.

Unsafe Movements

Be careful to avoid the following movements (they can slow down healing, create new pain, and even cause further injury):

- A slumped, head-forward posture
- Bending forward from the waist
- Twisting the spine to the point of strain
- Twisting the trunk and bending forward when coughing or sneezing or in activities such as vacuuming or lifting
- Anything that requires you to reach far and lift, such as heavy items on high shelves.

Picture Perfect Posture

I found a very helpful site that I suggest you visit and bookmark. To view photos that demonstrate proper body mechanics for many activities, see Tone Your Bones by the University of Alabama http://www.toneyourbones.org.

Travel Tips After Fracture

My husband, daughter, and I love to travel. My journeys across the globe have taught me a great deal. Here are some tips:

- During long trips by car stretch frequently. For example, when sitting keep the balls of your feet on the floor and raise your heels. Count to 10. Lower your heels back down and repeat 10 times. On a plane or train, take short walks down the aisle

- Travel with a small back cushion or Obus Forme back rest (confirm with the airline that you can bring this through security if traveling by air). Taxis and shuttle buses as well as road conditions vary across the world. Some have very few shock absorbers and it can be quite painful. I have experienced back pain from the run-down shuttle buses that transfer people from one area of the airport to another

- When booking hotels or apartments confirm that the bed has a firm mattress and, if possible, firm furniture (e.g., couches)

- Wear comfortable shoes with good support that have soles designed to prevent slipping

- Travel light. And when you do lift your bags—remember to maintain good body mechanics. I am still working on this!

- Invest in light luggage on wheels that roll easily

- When riding in an elevator, hold on to a railing and bend your knees slightly to prevent jolting your spine if the elevator lurches. Two years ago I was on my way to the third floor of an office building when the aged elevator lurched to a stop. I suffered in pain for weeks!

- Ask for help at the airport if you need it

- Car seat considerations are important to prevent pain and injury. Even in luxury cars they are often uncomfortable for people with back problems—especially those seats that are low and curved (as in sportier models). In a car, the seat is the most ergonomically important aspect to ensure comfort when you drive. Be sure that all parts of it provide you with decent support and that it has power adjustment controls for the seat, steering wheel, and the mirrors (after a fracture, reaching under to adjust the seat will be painful and might create new damage). Ensure that the seat is suitable in relation to your legs, hips, and back in particular, as car seats come in all different shapes and sizes.

Activities & Sports

The best activities and exercises are those that work the muscles harder than they would work normally. There is no way we can determine how much force it would take to cause a fracture in the spine so be vigilant and choose activities that are safe.

Keeping physically active is very important to my enjoyment of life, as well as my health goals. But I had to proceed with caution, as some of the activities and sports I enjoyed carried risks for people with fractures.

Proceed with Caution—Activities to Avoid or be Extremely Cautious

Consult with your doctor and physiotherapist on activities or sports that require you to bend, rotate or twist forcefully at the waist. If you decide to go ahead with them, ask your physiotherapist for advice on the correct body mechanics to minimize stress on you spine. The following list includes some of the worst offenders for putting pressure on the spine:

- **Golf.** Golfers bend over and twist repetitively, generating a tremendous amount of stress on the lower spine. There is a significant twisting force—much of the torque on the spine is generated in the windup and follow through of a long iron or wood shot

- **Tennis.** This high impact sport is considered to be beneficial for the prevention of osteoporosis but should be avoided if you already have the disease. There is risk of fracture from the torque on your back during jumps and swift direction shifts

- **Pilates and yoga.** Many of the poses and exercises require forward bending-flexion, side-bending, and rotation of the spine—all potentially damaging

- **Bowling and curling.** Both require forward bending

- **Cross-country skiing and skating.** There is force on the spine and the risk of falls

- **Exercise machines.** Cross country ski machines, rowing machines, stationary bicycles with moving handlebars, and any other machine that involves trunk rotation or forward bending can cause vertebral fractures in people with significant osteoporosis

- **Jogging, running, and jumping.** These are jarring to the spine and may cause new fractures, with enough impact.

Safer & Gentler Alternatives

You are probably thinking, "You gave me all the activities I shouldn't do. Now tell me what I can do!" Past and present physical activity has a protective effect on bone mineral density. I also feel happier and more energetic when involved in the following activities. I encourage you to find sports and disciplines that will be both suitably safe for your spine and enjoyable for you.

Tai Chi

Tai Chi, sometimes described as meditation in motion, can be a safe alternative to conventional exercises. A gentle and effective mind-body practice that originated in China as a martial art, Tai Chi consists of slow and gentle body moves while breathing deeply and meditating. It can help improve balance, slow bone loss, and relaxes the body and mind.

Nordic Walking

Nordic walking, a sport developed by cross country skiers as a summer training program, strengthens the muscles and benefits the bones of both the lower and upper body. Nordic walking uses two specially designed poles to work the upper body while walking. The poles are used by the arms to match each stride the person takes. It is low-stress and gives a total body workout. Because the poles assist with balance and on different surfaces, it is suitable for people of all ages and with varying abilities. Nordic Walking increases your heart rate, oxygen consumption, and caloric expenditure without increasing your perceived rate of exertion. You don't feel like you're working any harder but, in addition to working your legs, you're experiencing a full range of motion that engages the abs, arms, shoulders, upper chest, and back muscles. The poles provide additional stability and help reduce stress in the knees and other joints. Bone density can be increased through this sort of resistance training, and posture also improves through use of the proper technique and arm motion.

Because I was scared that I might inadvertently develop bad techniques that would hurt instead of help, I took a course with a qualified instructor who was very helpful and patient.

Swimming & Cycling

Swimming and cycling are terrific activities that work the heart and other muscles but since your body weight is supported by water or by a bicycle, you don't get the same bone-boosting benefits as weight-bearing exercises. You still require strength-training exercises. However, if you like to swim or cycle then continue to enjoy these activities along with your bone-building routine.

Be very cautious cycling as you don't want a fall that leads to a fracture. You may want to choose a bicycle that has a wider seat, back support, and is lower to the ground such as the Revive model I purchased (made by the Giant company). The Revive provides more comfort with a neutral riding position. It puts the rider in a more ergonomically correct position that takes pressure off the hands, shoulders, neck, back, and bottom.

Even after spinal fractures, you can stay active and take care of your bones!

CHAPTER 13

~

TO BRACE OR NOT TO BRACE

Soon after being diagnosed with spinal fractures, my orthopedic surgeon recommended that I see an orthotist and be fitted for a rigid back brace. Your doctor may also suggest this. These back supports are called orthotic devices and are designed to immobilize and support the spine. Bracing, like many treatments and therapies for the back, has its advocates and its opponents.

I believe my surgeon recommended a back brace because I was in constant, excruciating pain which made me open to trying anything to bring some relief.

It was not exactly fashionable! An upright molded piece in the rear curved to the shape of my spine and was inserted into a fabric cover. Three bands circled around the jacket and closed in front with Velcro straps. In my opinion, the back brace was helpful but I think I wore it too long. I should have discussed weaning myself off it earlier to reduce the loss of muscle in my abdominals and back. My muscles became so weak that when it was removed I could barely hold myself upright at the dinner table. In addition, I became psychologically dependent on the brace and felt fearful of injuring my spine if I wasn't wearing it.

Later, when seeing my endocrinologist for the first time, he expressed his views—he was clearly not in favour of bracing!

Although I experienced some muscle loss, the brace did provide me with enough support to get out of bed and function for short periods of time. So, although a brace may not be ideal, it might be better than resorting to bed rest to alleviate pain, as this can lead to further bone loss and other complications far worse than muscle loss.

This is yet another option that you need to discuss with your health care team and see if it is right for you.

What Is a Back Brace?

A back brace is a custom-made device that supports your back and restricts movement similar to the way a cast does when you break a bone.

What Does a Back Brace Do?

Back braces can offer a safe, non-invasive way to keep the spine in a neutral position, restrict motion (you can't bend forward), lessen the chance of another fracture, reduce the pressure on the spinal column, prevent further collapse of the bone, and allow healing of the fractures to take place.

Some people are more confident with the brace because they feel it is protecting their injured spine. Braces can bring pain relief through limiting the motion of the fractured vertebrae, taking pressure off the spinal column, and providing insulation and warmth just like a heating pad.

Steps to Getting a Back Brace

1. Your doctor refers you to an orthotist—an expert in making and modifying orthotic devices such as back braces.

2. The orthotist's goal is to design a brace that meets your doctor's requirements while considering your own needs for comfort. The aim of the orthotist should be to use as little bracing as possible to achieve the desired goals.

3. The orthotist is responsible for taking careful and precise measurements of you and supervising the making, fitting, and adjustment of the back brace. He or she should consider not only the location of the fracture but also your strength and flexibility when determining the type of closure for the brace (i.e., Velcro, buckles, hooks, or zippers). The brace will be custom fit to your body. After the brace is made, it may be necessary to have modifications made to ensure overall comfort.

4. The orthotist and your doctor should educate you in fitting and using the back brace (i.e., how long you should wear it each day and when you should start to reduce the number of hours in the brace). Most patients wear it in the day and remove it at bedtime.

5. Your doctor should monitor your progress, check to ensure your pain is subsiding, and use x-rays to ensure the vertebrae are stable and that the fracture is healing. These factors determine when it is time to stop using the brace.

What to Watch For

The brace can be helpful to take pressure off the unstable areas of the spine and the fractured vertebrae. However, if you wear the support all the time, it can weaken your abdominal and back muscles, as the brace is doing much of the work to hold up your spine and the muscles are doing very little.

Talk to your doctor and orthotist to determine how many hours the brace should be worn each day and how many weeks it will be necessary to use it. Typically, the brace is worn daily or while exercising or at times when pain relief is needed while your fractures are healing. Most fractures take two to three months to heal. Wear a cotton T-shirt underneath the brace so that the brace does not have direct contact with your skin—it's much more comfortable and helps avoid creating pressure sores.

Other Considerations

It is important to focus on weaning yourself off the brace gradually (in consultation with your doctor and physical therapist) once the fracture begins to heal. Start with gentle exercises to increase strength and endurance, increasing your activity level and improving your posture. You want to reduce the risk of psychological dependency on the brace.

Braces can be costly ($100 or more) so check to ensure whether your medical insurance, state, or province cover this cost.

Your doctor may or may not suggest a back brace. It will depend on the amount of support or stabilization required for the injury to your spinal column.

As with other treatment options, it is important to weigh both the benefit and cost of wearing a brace. If your doctor determines that your spine is unstable and/or your pain is so great that it is difficult to perform even simple daily tasks then bracing may be an option you should discuss with your doctor.

Brace or no brace, once your fractures have healed it is important to build resistance training into your exercise regime to improve muscle mass.

CHAPTER 14

~

SURGICAL OPTIONS

"Every year an estimated 1.4 million vertebral compression fractures that cause pain, disability and diminished quality of life come to clinical attention worldwide."

-Jan Va Meirhaeghe, MD, Orthopedic Surgeon
AZ Sint-Jan Hospital, Brugg, Oostende, Belgium

After spinal fracture(s), you may be one of the unfortunate patients who suffer intense, lasting pain that does not respond to medication, physical therapy or bracing. Sometimes the spine has collapsed to the point where it is unstable and breathing becomes difficult. Vertebroplasty and kyphoplasty are relatively new procedures—so recent that they were not options in Canada at the time that I fractured my spine—intended to treat pain and stabilize fractures. You and your doctor can investigate if these procedures are viable treatment options. This chapter provides an overview of information that may be helpful if you wish to talk to your doctor about either procedure.

Percutaneous Vertebroplasty
What Is it?

Percutaneous means a procedure performed through a small opening made in the skin. Vertebroplasty means fixing the vertebral body. The technique is most often performed by a specially trained radiologist and involves slowly inserting medical-grade acrylic cement through a special bone needle into the center of the collapsed spinal vertebra in order to stabilize and strengthen the crushed bone.

What it Is Intended to Do

The purpose of this procedure is to stabilize the fracture, reduce pain, and help you resume normal activity. The acrylic cement serves as an internal "cast." It can shorten recovery time from the fracture and help restore strength in the vertebra. Some experts believe that the pain relief is achieved through mechanical support and stability provided by the bone cement. Unfortunately, it does not restore the height or shape of the vertebra.

Most people with a compression fracture respond well to therapies such as bed rest, bracing, pain medication, and physical therapy. But a doctor may recommend this procedure for patients who fail to recover from spinal fractures, suffer from prolonged, severe pain, and remain immobile.

Kyphoplasty

What Is it?

Kyphoplasty is a modification of vertebroplasty. A pathway is made into the fractured vertebra. A small balloon is guided through the instrument into the vertebra. The balloon is then inflated to help raise the collapsed vertebra and restore it to its normal position. Then it is deflated and removed as the space created by the balloon is filled with quick-setting bone cement which stabilizes the fracture by acting as a "cast."

What it Is Intended to Do

The procedure stabilizes the fracture and restores the height of the compressed vertebra. It also reduces pain. This allows some compression fracture patients to reduce their pain medication and return to everyday activities such as walking and lifting with less pain.

What to Watch for

This procedure may not be suitable for men and women who:
- Have vertebral compression fractures that have healed and are responding to traditional therapies

- Have a fracture that is older than one year
- Have a fracture where the vertebra has collapsed to less than 30% of its normal height.

Health Canada posted a safety alert notice on their website (May 30, 2007) to hospitals on the complications associated with the use of bone cements used in vertebroplasty and kyphoplasty. They include but are not limited to:

- Death due to sudden blood pressure drop that may be related to the release of the bone cement into the bloodstream
- Leakage of the cement into the muscle and tissue surrounding the spine leading to neurological damage
- New fractures
- Pulmonary embolism (an air, blood, or cement clot that migrates to the lungs).

Other possible serious complications include heart attack, stroke, and paralysis. Also, as this procedure is relatively new, we do not know the long-term consequences of this cement in the vertebra.

Ideally, you should talk to patients with similar vertebral fractures who have gone through either of these surgeries, do some online investigation, and talk to your doctor before deciding to go through with either of these procedures. Keep in mind that there are risks, which vary by individual, associated with both operations.

The Canadian Family Physician site provides a list of and contact information for radiologists who perform vertebroplasty and kyphoplasty. There are many online sites with information on the procedures. Be wary of sites that praise the procedure (marketing!) and downplay the risks. I have provided some sites in the resources section to see visuals and videos of these procedures.

Conclusion

At this moment, the long-term data for outcomes of vertebroplasty or kyphoplasty do not exist. I do find it encouraging that there are new options to deal with the pain and spinal deformity caused by vertebral fractures that do not respond to traditional treatments.

Keep in mind that although vertebroplasty and kyphoplasty may reduce pain and strengthen the vertebra, they do not cure osteoporosis or prevent new fractures. You will still need to focus on building better bones through medications, adequate calcium and vitamin D, and physical activity.

CHAPTER 15

∼

Beyond Bones: Healing Emotions & Building Confidence

"Never underestimate your power to change yourself."
H. Jackson Brown Jr.

One fall night in 1991 I had a terrible car accident on the way to the theatre. It left me with a fractured foot, wrist, rib, and a burst fracture in a vertebra in my neck. For the first 24 hours after the accident the medical team tapped and tickled my hands and feet to ensure I still had sensation—they were worried that I might become paralyzed. Memories of this day returned a few years later when actor and activist Christopher Reeve became quadriplegic when he shattered his C-1 and C-2 vertebrae after landing head first after a fall from his horse.

I was young, single, successful, and often felt almost invincible driving what my father called "my fire engine red" Firebird. With the help of physiotherapy my body healed and I was back climbing the ladder of success at work in less than four months. After the initial shock of it all, the emotional scars from this healed quite quickly as I felt so fortunate to have averted paralysis in my lower limbs. A decade later, the emotional scars created by my diagnosis of osteoporosis and spinal fractures after my daughter's birth were far deeper and much more challenging to overcome.

Excerpts from my Diary
November 2001
 The pain is chronic and overwhelming. I experience physical pain as well as mental anguish because of my inability to take care of my one and only child. It hurts to sit,

stand, lie down, and even to roll over in bed. It is pretty hard to make any movement without the use of my spine!

Material things are no longer important. All I want is my health back. I was an independent, energetic person and now I am not capable of even being alone with my own daughter as I am unable to lift her or carry her. I whisper to my daughter—Mommy can't do much right now but I will make up for it when I am well. I envy my daughter Chanel's caregiver, Adoracion. Just yesterday when Chanel was hungry and started to cry, she did not reach for me to sooth her but to Adoracion to comfort her and wipe away the tears.

My husband has been unbelievably strong and patient through all this. He is used to being with a vibrant and independent woman and now I can't do anything for myself. It makes me so very sad. I often cry myself to sleep.

December 2001

Daylight is short and it is cold and icy so I am in the house most of the time. I begin to stay in bed longer in the mornings, take a longer nap in the afternoon, and go to bed earlier at night. Three very dear friends, Fiona, Peggy and Chris arrive at my home on December 10th to exchange Christmas gifts and decorate my home for the holidays. I have no real desire to celebrate Christmas. I make the motions for most of the evening but end up in tears. I explain that I am just overwhelmed by all the events and appointments over the last few months.

January 2002

My physician asks to speak to me alone without my husband. She asks me to consider taking an anti-depressant. At first I am surprised. Why me? I give this some thought. Another doctor had suggested this previously and so had my friend Peggy who was knowledgeable about the signs of depression. I agree to take a mild dosage. Months later I read how many patients suffering from osteoporosis or chronic pain sink into depression and sometimes need an anti-depressant.

April 2002

A turning point. The journey is getting better. I have a wonderful and supportive health care team including a smart and compassionate endocrinologist and a physiotherapist. I am doing my best to think positively and begin my journey to recovery. I get on the treadmill every day whether I want to or not. The mornings are good and the afternoons I am tired and sore. I make it around the block pushing my daughter in the jogger. My caregiver and I are elated! I try to be grateful and celebrate every moment.

Depression & Osteoporosis

I have learned that osteoporosis affects us emotionally as well as physically. Many studies support this and indicate that there is indeed a link between bone loss and depression. When treating the disease you have to mend both the body and soul.

Depression can come in many forms and some symptoms include:

- Sadness
- Anxiousness
- Pessimism
- Irritability
- Trouble sleeping
- Restlessness
- Changes in appetite
- Loss of interest in many things including sex.

Depression ranges from "the blues" to what Winston Churchill described as his "black dog," a feeling of hopelessness and despair.

After a fracture, many people experience anger and frustration because of the pain and physical limitations. We abandon activities and stay home more often to reduce the chance of another fracture. We feel anxiety and fear another fracture. We experience low self-esteem because of the change to our physiques the fractures cause. It resembles premature ageing. I often get asked if I am my daughter's grandmother!

Because acute osteoporosis and fractures are a huge physical blow and take up so much time and energy in terms of therapies, medical appointments and managing parts of daily life that used to be routine, the emotional trauma can be minimized or even ignored in the rush to deal with the physical aspects of getting well. But in my case it was a major hurdle. I couldn't even shower without my husband's help and I was completely dependent on others to take care of my first and only child. It was a very bitter pill to swallow. I lost almost two inches in height and the combination of pregnancy and fractures widened my waistline. I hardly recognized the body I saw in the mirror—I felt like I had aged a full decade in a mere three months. Then there was the never ending pain, the fear of another broken bone, and worries about what the future would bring. Anxiety set in and I kept wondering if the nightmare would ever end.

Seek Help

Studies have shown that only 30% of people with major depression seek help, partly because of the stigma and partly because they don't know it is a treatable condition. I can't think of anything more normal than becoming depressed after a spinal fracture and osteoporosis diagnosis. Pain, fatigue, fear about the future, a constant round of medical appointments, and working my derriere off in order to regain what I used to take for granted—not fun!

Depression is common and treatable. The sooner treatment begins the more effective it will be and the more likely you can prevent recurrences. There are several different types of antidepressant medications available today and they must be taken for several weeks before they begin to work.

If you think you are suffering from depression, see your doctor and get help for recovery. Your doctor will usually diagnose depression using signs, symptoms, family history, and possibly blood tests. There are many different treatment options available and it is important to know help is available and to take steps to get help. Your treatment choices will depend on your diagnosis severity and symptoms. See the Canadian Mental Health Association website for symptoms and visit Depressioncentre.net.

If you come from a "stiff upper lip" background that is suspicious of the notion of depression, be aware that several hard data studies show that depression is not only hard on the mind, it is hard on the body. Poor emotional health can weaken your body's immune system and slow down healing. A study conducted by Ohio State University researchers, published in the Archives of General Psychiatry in 2005, found that even mild depression can have long-term negative effects on health. As Dr. Robert Swenson, deputy head of psychiatry at the Ottawa Hospital General Campus, explained, "Our mind is linked to our brain, which is linked to our nervous and hormone systems, among other areas."

Depression itself can be bad for the bones, as are some of the drugs used to treat it. Long-term use of anti-depressants in the selective serotonin reuptake inhibitor (SSRIs) class can lead to bone loss. Other research points to depression itself as a source of endocrine changes that can damage bone. So your doctor will take this into account when prescribing an anti-depressant and treatment for your bone loss.

Anti-depressants are often the first treatment choice for adults with moderate or severe depression. Although anti-depressants may not cure depression, they can ease your symptoms and allow you to begin the healing process.

The first antidepressant you try may work fine. But if it doesn't relieve your symptoms, or it causes side effects that bother you, you may need to try another. All anti-depressants have pros and cons, and until you try one, you won't know exactly how well it will work for you. With persistence, you and your doctor should find one that works so that you can enjoy life more fully again. So don't give up. A number of anti-depressants are available, and chances are you'll be able to find one that works well for you.

I have experienced depression and I have come through it. There is a way to overcome these emotions. Medications and counseling help treat depression. It is a serious illness that can have profound consequences. Being sad, angry, or discouraged for a few weeks is normal when faced with a diagnosis of poor bone health. But if it persists it will impede your recovery, so let's look at ways to beat the blues.

After discussion with my doctor, I chose to take a mild antidepressant. The medication helped, but I think that using a collection of strategies—just as I did with my physical recovery—allowed me to emerge from my depression much faster. These techniques were also helpful with the mild recurrences of depression that the return of my pain would trigger.

A Chinese proverb states, "A journey of a thousand miles begins with a single step." When depression sets in we wonder how we will have the energy to attempt a single step, let alone one thousand miles.

Tools to Turn Around Your Mood

Many studies show that the most effective way to conquer depression combines medication, self-care, and therapy. Only a healthcare professional can diagnose depression. The following are simple and effective self-care tools that may complement what your doctor recommends if you are experiencing depression.

Breathe

Each day we take about 20,000 breaths. Breathe in and oxygen is delivered into our bloodstream through the lungs. Breathe out, and we get rid of waste gases like carbon dioxide. Breathing is something we don't think about and usually take for granted. What many people do not know is that fine-tuning your breathing can help calm and clear your mind, reduce tension and pain, and improve your mood and energy levels.

The diaphragm, the large flat muscle located between the bottom of the lungs and the top of the abdomen, plays a key role in healthy breathing. If your belly is relaxed the abdomen should fully expand when you breathe in. If belly muscles are tight, as a result of tension or poor posture, breathing becomes shallow and restricted. Also, many people unconsciously take shallow and shorter breaths when they are anxious.

To help you strengthen your diaphragm and use it correctly when you breathe, follow these steps:

1. Lie comfortably on your back on a firm bed. Relax your neck and shoulder muscles.

2. Place one hand on your tummy just below your rib cage and the other hand on your upper chest.

3. Inhale slowly and gently through your nose and begin expanding your abdomen. I emphasize the "gently" because even deep breathing hurt me at the acute fracture stage. The hand on your abdomen should rise higher than the one on your chest. This ensures that the diaphragm is pulling air into the bases of the lungs.

4. When your chest rises slightly, breathe out through your mouth slowly. Allow your abdomen to fall.

5. Continue exhaling. As your chest empties, allow the abdomen to begin to rise again. Repeat the cycle four more times for a total of five deep breaths.

In general, breathing out should take twice as long as breathing in. Once you feel comfortable with your ability to breathe into the abdomen, you won't need to keep your hands on your chest and abdomen.

Depression, hunched shoulders, and shallow breathing often go hand-in-hand. Breathing exercises such as this one can be done a few times a day or whenever you are experiencing pain, anxiety, or feeling low. It can help open up not only your chest but also your mind, body and spirit. It can improve your strength and energy. Be aware of your breathing throughout the day and take a moment to improve it using this exercise.

Meditate

In my 30s, like many Baby Boomers, I took various courses to learn how to cope with the stress that came from pressures of life and work. I enrolled in yoga and a Mindfulness Based Stress Reduction (MBSR) program which empowered participants to take an active role in the management of their health and wellness. After my fractures, yoga was not a viable option but the CDs from the

Mindfulness program with guided mindfulness meditation were and continue to be a source of support. Melodie Benger, an Ottawa-based MBSR instructor, describes mindfulness as follows: "Mindfulness is a way of learning to relate directly to whatever is happening in our life, a way of taking charge of our life, a way of doing something for yourself that no one else can do for us—consciously and systematically working with our own stress, pain, illness, and the challenges and demands of everyday life.

"Stress exists. Often the demands in our life seem greater than our available resources. Sometimes the way we react to stress creates more stress. Since our reaction to stress is usually automatic, we feel like we have no control. We may not be able to control our stressors but we can definitely control our reactions to stress. By becoming aware or mindful, we become more fully present in each moment. This awareness gives us the choice—to do what we have always done or to find a better way of responding to stress. Mindfulness practice helps you to see clearly with a broader perspective and helps you to connect with your own deep inner resources for coping."

Meditation is a practice that can be very confusing to most people. It brings to mind the image of a yogi sitting in the Lotus position with a beatific expression on his face. The main purpose of meditation is to still the mind and to become more in touch with your heart. There are many methods of meditation, and there are countless books, CDs and DVDs to choose from. There are many forms and breathing techniques and countless other tools in order to enable the mind to release thoughts. As there are many different kinds of people in the world, so there are many different kinds of meditation. To help beat the blues it's beneficial to try to find one that works for you.

A simple meditation:

1. Select a quiet comfortable place away from noise and distractions.

2. Sit with a neutral posture in a comfortable chair.

3. Close your eyes.

4. Breathe through your nose. Focus on your breath—cool air in, warm air out. A variation that may make things a little easier at the beginning is to count your breaths. Count up to four and then repeat, over and over.

5. If the mind wanders (mine does!) gently bring it back to the breath.

6. That's it. Start with a 5 to 10 minute meditation and work your way up to 15, 20, 30 minutes or more.

Progressive Muscle Relaxation

According to psychologist Mark Dombeck, who has focused his work on patients suffering from depression, negative emotion of any sort takes its toll on the body. Short, sharp emotions like anxiety and anger cause the body to tense up in preparation for action. Longer acting states like depression are associated with either tension or fatigue. These muscular states are not mere products of the negative emotion, but rather are part and parcel of it (think about a time you were angry and you can probably feel the muscles in your jaw and shoulders start to tighten). If you succeed in interrupting the muscular tension, you begin the process of defusing the negative emotion itself.

Just 10 minutes a day of a very simple technique called progressive muscle relaxation (PMR) can help reduce your anxiety and help you feel calm and relaxed. PMR teaches you to relax your muscles through a two-step process. First you deliberately focus on a certain muscle group and apply tension to that muscle group, and then you stop the tension and turn your attention to noticing how the muscles relax as the tension flows away. You should never feel pain while completing this exercise. Make the muscle tension deliberate yet gentle.

1. In a quiet room, lie down on your back in a comfortable position with your eyes closed, palms up and legs slightly apart (and a pillow under your knees if you need it to take the pressure off your lower back).

2. Relax and breathe deeply (as described earlier) for a minute or two. Breathe slowly and deeply throughout all the exercises. Do the exercises slowly starting from your feet and move up to the head.

3. Tense your toes. Curl your toes in your left foot hard toward the bed; hold for five seconds and relax; repeat with the right foot; then both feet together. Let all the tightness flow out of the tensed muscles. Exhale as you do this step. You should feel the muscles become loose and limp, as the tension flows out.

4. Tense your legs. Tense your left leg by pulling your toes towards you; hold for five seconds and then relax; repeat with the right leg; then both together and relax.

5. Tense your buttocks. Squeeze your buttocks together; hold for five seconds and relax. Repeat twice.

6. Tense your stomach; hold for five seconds and then relax. Repeat three times.

7. Tense your arms and shoulders. Shrug your shoulders up towards your ears; hold for five seconds and then relax. Repeat three times.

8. Tense your hands. Clench your right hand; hold for five seconds and relax; repeat with the left; then together.

9. Tense your face. Clench your jaw; hold for five seconds and then relax. Make a big frown on your face; hold for five seconds and relax.

10. Tense your entire body—every muscle you can from head to toe; hold for 10 seconds and relax. Let go of all the tension. Lie quietly for a minute or two.

11. Enjoy this relaxed state for a few minutes before getting up.

I find it helpful to listen to someone guide me through these steps. You can do the exercise yourself with relaxing music or you can buy or download progressive muscle relaxation exercises (or something very similar) to guide you through the steps.

Exercise

Even small amounts of exercise will benefit your mood—it triggers the production of endorphins (our natural pain relievers and mood elevators). These "natural" drugs are powerful stuff, perhaps hundreds of times more powerful than morphine. Exercise increases your energy and diverts your thoughts so you spend less time dwelling on your bones. It can be tough to start even a minimal exercise program because depression zaps your energy and limits motivation and drive—it's probably the last thing you feel like doing! Once you take that first step and begin to exercise you will become increasingly motivated by the benefits you receive. Completing even simple exercises gave me a sense of mastery over my condition and a sense of accomplishment that added a new dimension to my day. The bottom line is that most of us feel good after exercising.

See Chapter 11 for a list of exercises and techniques suitable for recovery from spinal fracture. Be sure to talk to your doctor and physiotherapist before beginning any exercise program.

An Image Consultant

"Fashion is illusion." *Yves St. Laurent*

Fractures affect the figure! The loss of height and curvature of my spine made me more compact and thickened my waist because the distance between my underarms and waist and my waist to my hips was less than it used to be. Clothes that used to look lovely no longer fit very well and shopping was frustrating. Some of my collared tops gaped; others still fit at the shoulders but were now too tight and pulled at the waist. Some jackets rode up in the back. Skirts and pants no longer hung properly. It might seem petty to someone who doesn't have osteoporosis, but the changes in how my clothes fit and how I looked when I caught a glimpse of myself in the mirror were a constant reminder of what I had lost.

When my husband asked me what I wanted for my birthday in 2005, I responded, "A consultation with an image consultant!" I explained how I felt about my "new, compact figure" and that I wanted an expert's opinion on how to enhance my sense of style with my new figure and shop more wisely. He graciously bought me the gift.

My stylist, Diane Craig, was kind and confident as she helped me build a wardrobe. We chose current fashions that fit my personal taste and flattered my new physique. Picking the right wardrobe helped me to accept what I cannot change about my body. It helped rebuild a positive self-image despite the consequences of my fractures. Through a figure and style analysis, I became more aware and more accepting of my body's proportions and learned secrets to enhance my overall appearance by selecting correct lines and designs. This was and continues to be one of my greatest investments in healing my emotional wounds and lifting my spirits. I believe in a saying I once heard—when you are grounded in your body your spirit soars!

If this is not in your budget there are other options. Work with department store personal shoppers (they are usually free). Or a local boutique may offer a staff member you trust to give you guidance on what is most suitable for your figure and tastes.

As my stylist stated, 95% of our body is covered with clothes and accessories so they have to say something! The following tips are gleaned from both Diane Craig and the National Osteoporosis Foundation's *Style Wise: a fashion guide for women with osteoporosis.*

1. Wear more black or solid dark colours as they can disguise a bulging tummy. Try a pair of black pants and black top. The solid top and bottom present a leaner image. Then add a sharp jacket for colour. If you wear black pants with a white top it will emphasize the waist. See it for yourself in a full-length mirror.

2. Overall, wear clothing that is loose, straight, or just slightly fitted.

3. Avoid horizontal stripes as they make you look wider; narrow vertical stripes give the illusion of slimness.

4. Jeweled, rounded, slight V, or soft cowl necklines work best.

5. Have tops outside of pants and not tucked in.

6. Add shoulder pads to compensate for sloping shoulders.

7. Avoid big and frilly cuffs that draw the eyes to the waist when the arms are by your side.

8. Wear dresses with an empire waist, dropped waist, or A-line.

9. Choose pants with a straight leg or a slight "boot cut" as they will make you appear taller and slimmer. Choose pants with a "clean front" meaning no pleats and, if possible, a side zipper to keep a smooth flow. Find pants with elasticized waistbands if others are uncomfortable.

10. Make good use of accessories, such as elegant costume jewelry, to highlight the face and neck and draw eyes up away from the tummy and shoulder area. If you aren't a "natural" shopper, staff in the smaller boutiques can be very attentive and helpful.

11. Wear scarves as they are one of the easiest ways to disguise shoulder and back curvature. A colourful or patterned scarf can help you feel great and update the look of an outfit. A scarf can fill a gaping collar or neckline. A bold scarf will also draw attention away from the shoulders and toward your face. A long scarf draped around the neck, flowing down the back, will give a longer profile.

12. Use compact, light women's backpacks to evenly distribute weight and leave hands free for balance. Many stores carry varieties that are far more fashionable than they used to be.

13. Wear flat or low-heeled comfortable shoes with rubber soles.

14. Avoid big wide belts at waist level as this breaks up the long line you are trying to achieve. Consider wearing a narrow or chain belt. Slung low on the hips it can actually lengthen the waistline. This looks especially good with a tunic top or top and bottom of a uniform colour. Or a wider belt below the hips if wearing a jacket that hangs down and covers the back. There are some fabulous belts that are both comfortable and fashionable with elastic in them.

15. Choose undergarments that fit properly and comfortably. Seek the help of knowledgeable sales staff. Look for specialty bras with adjustable crossed back straps or longer bra straps (or have a seamstress alter it by adding elastic extensions to the back

straps). Front hooks are easier for those who have restricted back movement. I have found that a poorly fitting bra can be a great source of discomfort. Focus on quality versus quantity; the right size and fit are much more important than a drawer full of ill-fitting bras.

16. Learn to choose the latest accessories and hottest fashion items that work with the classic pieces that flatter your figure.

17. Find a talented tailor to alter clothing so that clothes hang evenly and create a lengthening effect that minimizes the visual impact of the curvature in the spine.

18. Find retailers who also custom fit clothing for you. If you live in a smaller town where this is not an option, consider a yearly visit to a larger city—most retailers are happy to ship the clothes after they have been altered. Focus on quality versus quantity.

19. If possible, aim to keep a neutral posture and check it a few times each day. Slumping can cause your clothing to shift.

20. Highlight your assets! If you have beautiful eyes, choose clothing and accessories that draw attention to them. As challenging as it may be, aim to accept the changes to your body and love yourself just the way you are. Everyone looks more beautiful when they are confident.

Pamper & Reward Yourself

Keep your hair, make-up, skin, feet and nails in top condition. The more groomed and polished you are, the better you feel. In my darkest days of depression, my hair style, nails, and make-up were the last thing on my mind. I barely had enough initiative to shower and brush my teeth. Enhancing my appearance enhanced my mood. You may think this is superficial and silly, but looking good helps many of us feel good.

Bad hair days can be bad for your mood. For a boost, I turned to my trusted hair stylist for my long overdue highlights, a shampoo, a cut to best frame my face and a blow-dry. Going to a reputable salon allows you to sit back, be pampered from the minute you arrive, relax, enjoy a magazine, and imagine the scissors snip-snapping your troubles way. I think that the pampering and the pleasure I felt in my improved appearance (the "old" me was there again) was a reassurance that my situation could and would get better. Pamper yourself with a facial or pedicure or both! The treatments help heal the body and soul.

If you have accomplished a goal in your exercise program, reward yourself with a coffee out with a good friend, a new book, a dinner at your favourite restaurant or anything that is special to you. Or, invest in a new experience—many people are made happier by experiences than things.

Seek a Higher Power

Christian, Jewish, Buddhist, or whatever faith you practise, a belief in something bigger than you is a powerful resource that you can tap into as part of your healing process. For many, spirituality offers comfort in times of suffering and provides a message of hope. To quote Gabor Maté, the author of *When the Body Says No,* "Health rests on three pillars: the body, the psyche and the spiritual connection. To ignore any one of them is to invite imbalance and disease." The physiological explanation is that the meditative state that can occur while in prayer reduces emotional stress which, in turn, decreases blood pressure, relaxes muscles, reduces the secretion of stress hormones, and relieves insomnia. Also, prayer can have a positive effect on the immune system and help the body cope better with illness.

Humour

Children laugh 300 to 400 times each day whereas we adults take life much too seriously and laugh a mere 10 to 15 times a day. Laughter lowers blood pressure, reduces stress hormones, relieves physical tension, boosts the immune system, and releases endorphins, your body's natural painkillers. Humour changes our feelings, thoughts, behaviours, and biochemistry. We can develop and nurture humour to heal. We are all familiar with the great feeling after a deep belly laugh. Laughter can be a tremendous resource to heal a sad soul. As a start you may want to watch funny programs or movies on

TV or rent DVDs of your favourite comedies. Play fun games like Pictionary or charades. I found it helpful to spend time with friends who were naturally funny and who had a true zest for life. I knew they could distract my thoughts even for a short while. Playing with my daughter and her friends brightens my mood and brings out the kid in me!

Ask for Help

It took me a long time to learn to ask for help! Fill in the blank and repeat out loud "My back is really sore and even the simplest tasks are a challenge today so I am not up to _____ by myself. I need your help." To quote the late, amazing Gilda Radner, "It is important to realize that you have to take care of yourself because you cannot take care of anybody else until you do."

For Christmas 2009, I was to host 18 members of my family. Three weeks prior to the event I hurt my back and was in tremendous, unrelenting pain. I was chatting with my sister, Judy, when she urged, "Call in the troops, you can't do this on your own!" So I did! I contacted all the guests and asked them to bring a dish and then asked my other two sisters if they could come early to help set up the party room and stay late to help clean up. My guests, especially my sisters and their children, helped make the day special and enjoyable.

Beware of the Internet

The Internet is a double-edged sword. On the one hand it is a great resource to learn more about osteoporosis and how to manage the disease. On the other hand, it contains what I call "quack sites" filled with inaccurate information that can cause anxiety, fear, and hopelessness. Be selective and check to ensure the information comes from reputable sources such as the Scientific Advisory Board (SAC) of Osteoporosis Canada, the National Osteoporosis Foundation (US), or the International Osteoporosis Foundation. For example, the SAC may review a thousand studies on vitamin D before making a statement on daily recommended intake. Be especially careful of blogs with people giving advice on medications.

Take the information, summarize it, and discuss your concerns with your doctor. For example, enter the word "headache" into your search engine and you will come up with as many results for brain tumours as you will for caffeine withdrawal! The chances of you having a brain tumour are less than 1 in 10,000.

Let Go of the Anger

I reached a stage where I knew I had to let go of the anger that gripped me at having osteoporosis so young and the bitterness of developing significant bone loss while under doctors' close supervision during the eight weeks I was hospitalized. I had to get past that to get better. I felt that if I did not manage it, it would manage me. I needed to focus my energy on more important things. I realized I had to take ownership of my own health, educate myself about the condition, and pay attention to my treatments, even if it means asking doctors uncomfortable questions. I came to the realization that everyone is really just doing their best. I mean, nobody comes to work in the medical field and says "Gee, we're going to let this patient fall through the cracks."

I also replayed the night I tried to lift my daughter out of the crib over and over again—the night I must have sustained some spinal fractures. I needed tools to break these unhealthy and destructive thought patterns so that I could regain my strength and live an active life again.

Affirmations

Affirmations and visualization use mental exercises to change physical health. Setting goals and visualizing yourself achieving them are key to recovery. Creating a mental image of what you want to happen and how you want to feel is key to the road to recovery. Athletes do this to enhance their performance.

While recovering, I knew I needed to stop my gloomy, hurtful "self-talk." One of the features of depression is that it distorts thinking which is why incantations and affirmations can be helpful to stop those damaging thoughts.

When overwhelmed with pain, it was easy to assume and believe that I was never going to get better again or be able to take care of my daughter and enjoy being a wife and mother again. There came a time when I knew I needed to say and do things to halt these negative thoughts, even just temporarily. At first I did not truly believe some of my affirmations but the more I repeated them aloud the more I was convinced that I was on the road to recovery. It may sound silly or simplistic, but research shows that mental and emotional expectations can influence medical outcomes.

I contacted a very dear friend, Sandra Perron, Canada's first female infantry officer, who has overcome many challenges thrown her way. While serving in the armed forces, she was beaten and tied barefoot to a tree during a 1992 military training exercise and the horrific picture graced many Canadian newspapers and TV stations. Sandra left the army in 1996 and later became the chair of a nine-member board to review policies and interview all ranks of army personnel to make recommendations to the Defence Minister. Sandra stated in one newspaper article: "Some of my own challenges have helped me understand the heart of integration issues. I've thought long and hard about this appointment and I thought there's no way God has made me go through all this not to help."

I contacted Sandra because she was an inspiration to me. She came to my home with visualization tapes in hand. She shared how they might be helpful in setting achievable goals and managing my thoughts and visualizing what I want to achieve. When I got on the treadmill each day I would listen to those tapes over and over again.

Affirmations are positive statements about you and your health. They are spoken out loud in the first person in the present tense. Visualization or guided imagery is mobilizing the imagination to promote physical and emotional healing.

I also listened to CDs by Anthony Robbins, who is a master at visualization and affirmations. His program taught me to spend time each day thinking about what I am grateful for—my family, my friends, and the small improvements in my health. I would visualize my body healing, and my bones and muscles getting stronger and repeat simple incantations—words that are repeated to achieve a desired effect—such as:

"I am getting healthier and stronger every day."

"My back is healing."

"My bones and muscles are getting stronger every day."

"I feel great!"

Nutrition

You have heard the old expression "You are what you eat." Many people don't realize how poor eating habits affect their moods. Our brain uses a lot of calories and nutrients as part of its daily process. Emotions are generated in the physical brain. When we don't give the brain an adequate supply of nutrients at the right time (even your car needs gas, oil, radiator fluid, and brake fluid at regular times or it breaks down), our thinking and our emotions suffer. This is even truer when facing a major challenge like long-term pain and recovery from spinal fracture.

There are many reasons why we might deprive ourselves of the nutrients we need:

- The convenience of fast food

- Fat, sugar, and salt taste good to most of us

- Don't like cooking

- Prefer coffee and a donut to a nourishing breakfast

- An eating disorder.

There are hundreds of books that provide explanations and a bewildering list of "right" ways to eat. I use *Canada's Food Guide* for ways to achieve a balanced diet and maintain healthy eating habits that work for me (it's free and was created by dozens of nutritionists and scientists working together). Eating the amount and type of food recommended and following the tips included in *Canada's Food Guide* helps meet my needs for vitamins, minerals and other nutrients and contributes to my overall health and vitality.

Up to 68% of depressed people have a nutritional deficiency (Dr. Melvin Werbach, UCLA School of Medicine). Depression tends to alter your appetite. In addition to making healthy food choices, vitamins and supplements are often valuable in providing balanced material we need to produce crucial brain chemicals, including serotonin.

Deficiencies in folate (the synthetic form in supplements is called folic acid), vitamin B12 and vitamin B6 are common nutritional issues associated with depression. To ensure your nutritional needs are met in these areas include foods rich in these vitamins or consult your doctor regarding supplements (not all supplements are created equal). The best sources of B6 are high-protein foods like meat, fish and chicken (*Leslie Beck's Nutrition Guide for Women*). Other good sources include whole grains, bananas, and potatoes. The best sources for folate include spinach, artichokes, asparagus, lentils, dried peas and beans, and orange juice. Foods containing vitamin B12 include meat, fish, poultry, dairy products, eggs, and fortified soy and rice beverages.

Julia Ross, author of *The Mood Cure*, recommends reducing your caffeine, aspartame, and fast food intake—all of which can inhibit the production of serotonin, the natural chemical in your body that has a calming and relaxing effect.

(I delve more deeply into nutrition in Chapter 16).

Beat the Blues while Bonding with Peers

It is very common to withdraw from other people when you are depressed—unfortunately, loneliness can deepen depression. Social contact, often the last thing you feel like reaching for, can help lift you out of the dark moods. If anxiety and fear have immobilized you, talk to someone who has been there and struggled with the same issues. Joining an osteoporosis support group gives you access to current, accurate information.

It gives you an opportunity to share your experiences, listen to others' experiences, help each other understand the choices, learn more about the physical and emotional issues related to osteoporosis, and empower one another to be informed patients. Support groups may communicate through newsletters, formal meetings, or through internet sites. A group effort can make changes in lifestyle, improving and promoting coping skills, and stress reduction easier to access. Change is tough and it helps to know others are coping with similar issues.

A group process with female peers can help eliminate a sense of isolation, reduce depression, and increase the odds that you will take the necessary steps to improve well-being. Researchers have reported that just having one "significant" confidant can improve overall health and well-being (Brown 1975, et al. and Broadhead 1983, et al.). Hearing another person's experience provides comfort and encouragement that things will get better for you.

My physiotherapist was able to connect me with a woman who was also in her 40's when she suffered spinal fractures. It gave me hope to talk to someone who had faced the same challenges and was now leading an active life.

As the chairwoman of the Ottawa Chapter of Osteoporosis Canada I was instrumental in launching the Strong Bones Peer Support Group in Ottawa in 2008 and it has been a very rewarding experience. I am a firm believer in the value of self-help groups as an excellent source of support, advice, strength, and hope for those living with osteoporosis. To find a support group near you contact Osteoporosis Canada or the National Osteoporosis Foundation or the osteoporosis organization in your country.

Sex & Fracture

Sexuality is a joyful part of life for many of us. After a spinal fracture, pain, sense of fragility, and fear of new injury can lead to changes in the bedroom. The fun and the intimacy of sex is yet another thing that seems to have been taken away—and it may create even more of a sense of isolation from our spouse. This painful loss can contribute towards sinking into depression.

Let me reassure you—you can enjoy a fulfilling sex life after fractures, although you may have to make a few changes in technique and positions.

Soon after the diagnosis of the broken bones in my back, I remember my physician asking me the method of birth control I was using. My response?

"Fractures!"

Sexual intimacy was the absolute last thing on my mind when depressed and in pain. But once I began to feel stronger my desires returned. On one hand I wanted to experience that intimacy again and on the other hand I was anxious about injuring my back.

It is important for both you and your partner to be patient, have an open mind, communicate, and be willing to explore. You may need to find different sexual positions that will be comfortable for each of you and satisfy you both. Although your sexual experiences may be different than they were before your fractures, they can still be satisfying. And sometimes even better than before your back injury!

Because both patient and health care provider usually feel a bit uncomfortable about this topic, the issue of sex after fracture may not be raised in the doctor's office. I think it is important to bring it up. If your doctor is too uncomfortable to discuss it or simply doesn't have information, ask for a reference to someone who can help you. Sex is an important part of human relationships and it is worth putting a bit of investigation into finding out how it can become part of your life again.

I found that the book *Your Aching Back* (Augustus A. White III, MD) gives useful descriptions and diagrams on how to make love with a back problem. He suggests you try a "practice run." He refers to this as making love with the air, as you slowly try sexual manoeuvres without your partner. If there is no pain, try it again with the air a little more vigorously and gradually move to gentle intercourse with your partner. The key is to find sexual intimacy that leads to far more pleasure than pain and eventually no pain at all. And don't forget that the endorphins produced during sex are great natural pain killers and mood elevators!

Communicating with Family & Friends

Osteoporosis is more than unhealthy bones. The emotional side of the disease can be overwhelming and it affects family and extended family. Having long-term pain, depression, or the diagnosis of a chronic disease can put a strain on all your relationships. During the acute stages of my fractures, when the pain was unrelenting, I struggled with friends and family. Many would call and say "Are you feeling better today?" And actually the pain was worse… and some days I felt like I was sliding into a black pit of despair. If I revealed that I was not feeling great there was often silence on the other end of the phone. They really did not know what to say as my situation dragged on for days, then weeks, and then months. I truly appreciated those phone calls but found it difficult to express exactly how I felt. I am a very social person but at that time in my life I really did not want to see or talk to many people. I was so fortunate to have family and friends who truly rallied and continued to support me. What I have learned from this experience is how to deal with others who are ill. Here are a few suggestions of actions and words that I found most helpful:

- Say: "I am sorry for your pain"
- Try to listen more and acknowledge feelings and not give advice or tell people how to feel
- Drop off a meal or snacks
- Send a card and let them know you are thinking about them
- Offer to drive them to an appointment or baby sit
- Buy trashy, entertaining magazines and drop them off
- Keep visits short
- Offer to take them out somewhere but call first. Don't drop by unexpectedly just in case the person is having a bad day
- Don't say "You'll be fine"
- Be supportive and don't be offended by unanswered calls.

Volunteer

When we share our time and talents we improve lives, we connect with others, and we transform our own life. A growing body of research shows that volunteering provides social benefits and health benefits. Those who volunteer later in life have greater functional ability and lower rates of depression than those who do not volunteer.

Once I felt strong enough, I contacted Osteoporosis Canada as I wanted to help others struggling with osteoporosis. With an Executive Master of Business Administration from Queen's University, I knew I had skills to offer, and now I had the personal motivation to contribute. I was and still am passionate about wanting to educate people on how to prevent and manage the disease. In addition, you can be a voice for others too frail to volunteer and help improve access to medication, BMD tests, and health care.

As I have stated before, osteoporosis can be 3D—depressing, debilitating, and devastating. But it does not have to be. With the right information, support and care, you can regain and maintain a healthy lifestyle and manage the disease.

Get the Sleep You Need

Sleep is often the first to go when a person is in pain and/or depressed. A few restless nights is okay but it soon becomes detrimental to your physical and emotional health. Treating insomnia can be a stepping stone to better health. Try to discover consistent bedtime rituals that relax you and allow you to have a good night's sleep. Aim to go to bed at the same time each night and awake at the same time each morning.

Everybody's needs are different. The range of time people sleep varies from 3 to 10 hours. As a general rule of thumb, 5 to 6 hours of sleep is probably a minimum. Below this your performance when driving, at work, etc., will be affected. Most people need between 7 and 8 hours sleep a night to feel refreshed. Here are some tips:

- Make your bedroom a cozy, peaceful place—relaxing décor and bedding
- Make sure you have a supportive mattress and pillow placement to minimize spine pain
- Make sure the room temperature is comfortable
- Listen to calming music
- Keep the room dark and quiet
- Pray, meditate, deep breathe, or try progressive relaxation

- Avoid heavy meals two hours before bedtime
- Avoid food and beverages that contain caffeine in the evening.

A Partner's Perspective

I asked my husband to share his suggestions from having lived through my dark days with me.

His first response was "That period is a blur to me." Upon reflecting for a few minutes he came up with some valuable suggestions. Focus on one day at a time and remember that each day is better than the last. As a partner, try to find time for yourself and time to exercise. Be a good listener and keep encouraging your partner even in her darkest moments. Always focus on the progress even if it is baby steps forward. Focus on the next thing you can do to take a step forward. Keep trying new tools and never quit. If one tool doesn't work try another to discover how to make life easier. For example, if meditation is not your thing then try progressive relaxation or other tools that work for you.

Our daughter was born 13 days after September 11, 2001—a day that changed the world. My husband had many challenges at the time as he was newly appointed as a senior bureaucrat at Citizenship and Immigration Canada. He said it was important for a partner to keep a balance and figure out what you are capable of doing and where you need help. Draw on family and friends to help. It is easy to isolate yourself from others. He said if he plotted the journey on a curve it would look like this—an initial sharp downward trend at the acute stage of the fractures; then after the shock of the diagnosis, an even sharper dive; then a plateau as reality sets in and we develop ways to move forward; then a turning point where we made changes in the home to help with recovery and now progress begins; then—once I began treatment with a mild anti-depressant, started exercising, and using the other tools in this chapter—he saw a sharp and steady curve upwards.

For the Doubter

You may be deeply skeptical about some of the techniques I used to help my mental and emotional recovery—I had my own doubts. I only tried some of these methods because I was at the end of my rope. But they helped me to get better and move towards a life that is enjoyable. I encourage you to try them—give it 28 days and see if you feel an improvement in your quality of life. You may feel more comfortable if you understand that, while many of these methods are talked about in spiritual terms, they do alter brain and body chemistry in a way that is measurable and promotes better moods and faster healing.

CHAPTER 16

~

YOUR BODY'S
BEST FRIEND: NUTRITION

I f you Google "nutrition and osteoporosis" a bewildering number of results will come up—some selling the latest "miracle" product, some with a mile-long list of forbidden items. I am an advocate of moderation, something my father, who lived to be 90, always believed. I am not going to tell you to toss your Starbuck's or give up wine. If we eat well by choosing wisely from a variety of food groups we can treat ourselves. In this chapter I hope to dispel some myths and share some of the information about nutrients that will help you live well with osteoporosis.

I was asked by my life wellness coach to review my diet to assess how I was doing in terms of contributing to my overall health and vitality. I recorded my food and beverage intake for two weekdays and two weekend days. Yikes! This was a real eye opener for me. I was so focused on my dairy and vitamin D intake that I neglected other important nutrients that promote health and vitality. This exercise gave me the incentive to explore nutrients further and write this chapter.

Food nourishes the body and gives us energy to get through the day. Healthy eating is fundamental to good health and is important in reducing the risk of many chronic diseases. Also, it plays a role in helping manage any chronic disease—including osteoporosis. In the following pages, I share what I have learned about the nutrients and eating habits that can help build bone health.

Calcium: the Best Bone Builder

Calcium is nothing short of amazing! It is needed for the formation and maintenance of bones and the development of teeth and healthy gums. It is necessary for blood clotting, stabilizes many body functions, and is thought to help prevent bowel cancer.

It has a natural calming and tranquilizing effect and is necessary for maintaining a regular heartbeat and the transmission of nerve impulses. It helps with lowering cholesterol, muscular growth and the prevention of muscle cramps. Furthermore it also helps with protein structuring in DNA and RNA. It provides energy, breaks down fats, maintains proper cell membrane permeability, aids in neuromuscular activity and helps to keep the skin healthy. About 99% of our calcium is found in our bones and teeth—the rest circulates in the blood and cells. If you consume too little calcium, the body pulls it out of the bones, which can create weak, fragile bones.

How Much Calcium Do We Need To Consume Every Day?

According to Osteoporosis Canada and the National Osteoporosis Foundation (US):

Table 16.1

Age	Daily calcium requirement
4 to 8	800 mg
9 to 18	1300 mg
19 to 50	1000 mg
50+	1200 mg
pregnant or lactating women 18+	1000 mg

Unfortunately, many North American women aren't getting enough calcium.

Calcium absorption is as high as 60% in infants and young children, who need substantial amounts to build bone. Absorption decreases to about 20% in adulthood and continues to decrease as people age, which is why higher calcium intakes are recommended for men and women over 50 years old.

The amount of calcium in a food is not the only consideration. We must be able to absorb it so that our bones and whole body benefit from it. Generally speaking, plant foods contain substances that bind to calcium and make it harder for us to absorb it.

I find it difficult to consume my daily requirement of calcium in the form of food. The most efficient way for my family and me to get calcium is through dairy products like milk, yogurt, and cheese. In lieu of plain coffee, I drink a Starbucks latté in the morning. It is my treat!

I am not going to get into debate about dairy—a book in itself! I am going to share what I know and you can decide whether you want to include dairy in your diet.

One very important fact that I learned is that the amount of calcium you absorb from the foods you eat depends not only on how much calcium is in the food, but on how easily it's absorbed (bioavailability). Many researchers say that the best bet for getting calcium is from dairy products like milk, yogurt, and cheese because they are high in calcium and the type of calcium they contain is easily absorbed by the body.

It is a challenge to meet calcium recommendations from plant sources like green vegetables, legumes, nuts, and seeds so it is especially important to rely on sources that contain well-absorbed calcium. (See Tables on pages 190 and 191 for some comparisons.)

Four factors are important in determining how much calcium we obtain and retain from foods.

1. The amount of calcium in the serving of food.
2. How easily the calcium is absorbed (bioavailability).
3. Eating foods that interfere with calcium absorption and cause it to be lost in the urine. e.g., excess coffee and excess salt.
4. Getting enough vitamin D to promote absorption.

Milk and milk products are rich in protein, calcium, riboflavin and vitamin B12—nutrients essential to good health. It is difficult to obtain your daily requirements of calcium and vitamin D without consuming milk or milk products. Studies show that people who drink more milk not only get more calcium, but also get significantly more magnesium, potassium, zinc, iron, vitamin A, riboflavin, and folate.

Canada's Food Guide recommends drinking 3 cups (500 mL) of milk every day or milk alternatives such as yogurt or a fortified soy beverage.

According to Health Canada, fortified soy beverages, although not identical to cow's milk, are a nutritionally adequate alternative. They are suitable beverages for those who cannot or do not drink milk.

If you are lactose intolerant or vegan, you can, with a bit of work, get ample calcium in your diet. See Table 16.3 (Page 191) for some non-dairy foods that contain calcium that is well absorbed.

Cutting Through the Confusion about Calcium Supplements.

If you find it difficult to obtain the recommended amounts of calcium (e.g., have high calcium needs and a small appetite) through diet alone, a combination of foods rich in calcium and calcium supplements is a good strategy. Calcium supplements come as tablets, capsules, or liquids containing the mineral calcium from a non-food source.

The market for calcium supplements is huge, and slick manufacturers will say anything to get you to try their product. Not all calcium compounds are created equal. Here are some tips to choosing a calcium supplement from Osteoporosis Canada:

- Check the amount of elemental calcium on the product label as this is the figure used to calculate your true daily intake, e.g., 500 mg of elemental calcium in each 1250 mg tablet of a brand of calcium carbonate

- The most expensive preparations are not necessarily the best. Costs will vary among brand name products and similar generic supplements. Prices also vary with the amount of elemental calcium per tablet. Compare brands and prices

- For some, calcium supplements may cause stomach upset, constipation, or nausea. Try different brands or forms, e.g., chewable or effervescent tablets, to find a suitable product for you.

The best two sources of calcium in a supplement are calcium carbonate and calcium citrate.

How to take a supplement:

1. Take calcium carbonate with food or immediately after eating. It is absorbed more effectively when there is food in the stomach. Calcium citrate, calcium lactate, and calcium gluconate are well absorbed at any time.

2. Take calcium supplements with plenty of water.

3. Take no more than 500 mg of elemental calcium at one time.

4. Talk to your doctor and pharmacist about possible interactions with other medications you take.

Calcium citrate is recommended for women over the age of 50, as the amount of calcium carbonate you absorb depends on how much stomach acid is present. As people age the stomach produces less acid. Because of this, calcium citrate is a better choice for people over the age of 50 as it is one of the most absorbable forms of calcium.

Table 16.2: Comparison of sources of absorbable calcium with milk

Food	Serving Size g	Calcium content mg	Fractional absorption %	Estimated absorbable calcium mg
Milk	240	300	32	96
Fortified soy beverage	240	300	23	55
Red beans	172	40	24	10
Bok choy	85	79	54	43
Broccoli	71	35	61	21
Cheddar cheese	42	303	32	97
Chinese cabbage	85	239	40	95
Juice with calcium	240	300	52	156
Kale	85	61	50	30
Spinach	85	115	5	6
Sweet potatoes	164	44	22	9
Rhubarb	120	174	9	10
Tofu with calcium	126	258	31	80
Yogurt	240	300	32	96

(*Summarized from The American Journal of Clinical Nutrition, Comparison of sources of absorbable calcium with milk, www.ajcn.org/cgi/content/full/70/3/543S/ T2 and Dairy Nutrition, Calcium and Bioavailability www.dairynutrition.ca/nutrients-in-milk-products/calcium/calcium-and-bioavailability*)

A food's value as a source of calcium is dependent on two things: how much calcium it actually contains (its absolute content) and its bioavailability factor. We've already seen that milk and milk products are the champions when it comes to providing large portions of calcium that our body easily absorbs. The following chart (created by Helen Bishop MacDonald) shows the quantity of 10 types of non-milk foods you would need to eat in order to absorb the same amount of calcium in 1 cup of milk.

Table 16.3

Food	Approximate serving Size equivalent to I cup (250 ml of milk)
Almonds	¾ cup (175 ml)
Chickpeas cooked	3 ¾ cups (875 ml)
Salmon, pink, canned with bones	¾ of a 213 g can
Salmon, sockeye, canned, with bones	¾ of a 213 g can
Sardines, canned with bones	7 medium (83 g)
Sesame seeds	1 ¾ cups (425 ml)
Soybeans, cooked	1 ¾ cups (425 ml)
Soy beverage	31 ½ cups (7.875 L)
Soy beverage, fortified	1 cup (250 ml)
Tofu, regular, processed with calcium sulfate	2/3 cup (200 g)

A to Z: Bones Need More than Calcium

Many of us have a fuzzy idea of "healthy" when it comes to food. And our minds help trick us—studies have shown we'll remember eating an apple (healthy) and forget the two donuts (not so healthy). The Canada Food Guide webpage and the US Department of Agriculture Food Pyramid tell you everything you need to know about the basics of a balanced diet that provides the nutrients our bodies need to function at their best. The British version is even simpler; the Eatwell Plate (www.eatwell.gov.uk) shows you the types of food and portions that make up a healthy plate. (The resource section on this chapter also lists books by Leslie Beck and Helen Bishop MacDonald that I found very helpful.)

The health profession has done a good job of promoting the message that calcium is necessary for healthy bones. But we aren't so clear about the fact that calcium cannot do its critical work alone. To do its job effectively, it needs the support of a bone-building team of many nutrients and minerals. These 26 key nutrients and minerals affect your overall health and many can influence and contribute to your bone quality and density. Where applicable, I have included the recommended dietary allowances (RDA) from Health Canada for women aged 50.

A cautionary note—these are reference values for normal, healthy individuals eating a typical North American diet. Osteoporosis, other health issues, and your lifestyle mean that you should talk to your doctor about tailoring specific nutrients to meet your needs.

A Is for Vitamin A

Vitamin A helps promote vision, growth, and bone development. It helps boost the immune system, protect against infection, and keep the skin healthy. Two of the most common sources of vitamin A are retinol and beta-carotene. Retinol is found in animal foods such as liver, eggs, and fatty fish. It also can be found in many fortified foods, such as fortified milk, cheese, breakfast cereals, and in dietary supplements. Beta-carotene is found naturally in mostly bright orange and dark green fruits and vegetables. The best sources of vitamin A include: carrots, winter squash, sweet potatoes, spinach, broccoli, romaine lettuce, apricots, peaches, mango, and cantaloupe. While vitamin A is crucial for healthy bones, some studies conclude that too much vitamin A is linked to bone loss and hip fracture. The recommended dietary allowance (RDA) of vitamin A for women is 2330 International Units (IU) and it is not advisable to take over 10,000 UI daily.

B Is for Vitamin B6

Vitamin B6 affects both physical and mental health and is involved in more bodily functions than any other single nutrient. Among other roles, vitamin B6 is involved in the production of antibodies and the creation of serotonin, the brain chemical that has a calming and relaxing effect. Food sources of B6 are high-protein foods like meat, fish, poultry, whole grains, bananas, and potatoes. The RDA for women is 1.5 milligrams (mg). One banana is .7 mg, or almost half the daily RDA.

C Is for Vitamin C

Vitamin C is responsible for more than 100 functions in the body ranging from boosting the immune system to reducing the risk of cataracts, colon cancer, and heart disease. A primary function of vitamin C is the manufacture of collagen, the main protein substance in the body. Collagen fibers keep bones and blood vessels strong, and help to anchor our teeth to our gums. Collagen is also required for the repair of blood vessels, bruises, and broken bones.

We know that the best sources of vitamin C are citrus fruits and their juices. Fruits high in vitamin C content include oranges, lemons, peaches, strawberries, kiwis, and grapefruit. A cup of sliced strawberries provides 140% of the RDA for vitamin C. Foods that also contain high quantities of vitamin C include broccoli, cauliflower, red pepper, tomatoes and potatoes. The RDA for women is 75 mg—one orange is 70 mg. The upper limit is 2000 mg.

D Is for Vitamin D

Most women are aware that calcium is essential to good bone health but few are aware that vitamin D is also critical to absorb calcium.

Vitamin D is vital to our bones, muscles and body, especially in children and the elderly. According to the Canadian Cancer Society, there is growing evidence that vitamin D may reduce the risk of some types of cancer, particularly colorectal and breast cancers. Experts are now concerned that many people are not getting enough vitamin D.

Calcium and vitamin D have been called the dynamic duo that need each other to boost bone health. Without vitamin D, our bodies can't use calcium properly and vice versa. Vitamin D enhances the ability of calcium to be absorbed into the osteoblast cells of the bones. We get vitamin D from our diet (or supplements) and sun exposure. Special cells in our skin produce vitamin D when they're activated by the ultraviolet rays of the sun. Vitamin D not only helps with calcium absorption, it also aids in the biomechanical process by which calcium turns into bone. Too little vitamin D can cause calcium and phosphorus levels in the blood to decrease, leading to calcium being leached out of the bones to help maintain stable blood levels.

Research has shown that most Canadians are vitamin D deficient at some point during each year for four reasons:

1.   As we age, our skin becomes less efficient at producing vitamin D from sunlight.

2.   Canada's northern climate means UVB levels in sunlight are too weak 4 to 6 months of the year to make any vitamin D naturally.

3.   Sunscreen use shields us from the sun and the production of vitamin D.

4.   Very few foods contain vitamin D. Significant sources include salmon, sardines, and fortified milk, eggs, and margarine.

Osteoporosis Canada (OC) and the National Osteoporosis Foundation (US) recommend a daily vitamin D intake of:

Table 16.4

Age	OC Daily intake in international units (IU)	NOF Daily intake in international units (IU)
Men and women (under age 50)without osteoporosis or conditions affecting vitamin D absorption	400-1000 IU	400-800 IU
Men and women (age 50+)	800-2000 IU	800-1000 IU

As it's almost impossible to get enough vitamin D from diet alone (8 ounces of vitamin D fortified milk provides 100 IU, requiring you to drink 4 to 10 cups of milk each day to hit your target), most health care professionals recommend that adults consider taking a vitamin D supplement. Talk to your doctor about taking 1000 international units (IU) a day during fall and winter months.

According to the NOF, previous research suggested that vitamin D3 (called cholecalciferol) was a better choice than vitamin D2 (called ergocalciferol). However, more recent studies show that vitamin D3 and vitamin D2 are equally good for bone health. In Canada, OC still recommends vitamin D3.

E Is for Vitamin E

Vitamin E, a powerful antioxidant, can help reduce blood pressure, and may help prevent certain cancers, heart disease, dementia and cataracts. Sources include wheat germ, nuts, seeds, vegetable oils, and whole grains. It may be challenging to meet the RDA for women of 15 IU, as two tablespoons of wheat germ is 4 IU. The upper limit is 1000 IU of natural vitamin E.

F Is for Folate (Vitamin B9) & Vitamin B12

Vitamin B9, called folate when it occurs naturally in foods, is needed for energy production, the formation of red blood cells, and lifelong bone repair and bone-building. It can help prevent heart disease, anxiety, depression, and reduce the risk of colon cancer. The best food sources of vitamin B9 include spinach, artichokes, avocado, asparagus, lentils, leafy greens, and orange juice. The RDA for women is 400 micrograms (mcg) (e.g., 1 cup of orange juice provides 115 mcg).

Folate and vitamin B12 work closely together in the body.

Without enough vitamin B12, the osteoblasts can't do their job and your body is unable to use folate. Vitamin B12 is required for proper digestion, absorption of food, and nerve function. Food sources for B12 include meat, fish, poultry, dairy products, eggs, fortified soy and rice milk, and fortified cereals. The RDA for women is 2.4 mcg (e.g., 1 cup of milk provides .9 mcg).

G Is for Grain Products

Grains are the seeds of plants such as wheat, rice, oats, barley, corn, wild rice, and rye, as well as pseudocereals like quinoa and buckwheat. Grains can be either whole (pretty much as they were picked) or refined (parts removed and/or bleached).

Canada's Food Guide (2007) recommends that women have six grain portions a day and that you make at least half of your grain product choices whole grain each day—do check the portion sizes as a large bagel, for example, can contain four portions of grain. Whole grains are a source of fibre and are usually low in fat. A diet rich in whole grains has been shown to have a number of health benefits and may help reduce your risk of heart disease. Bottom line: limit refined grains such as white bread and go for the whole grains instead.

H Is for Health Canada

Health Canada, through the *Eating Well with Canada's Food Guide* (2007), educates and helps people follow a healthy diet by guiding food selection. The guide translates the science of nutrient requirements into a practical pattern of food choices, incorporating variety and flexibility. I encourage you to visit the site (www.hc-sc.gc.ca/fn-an/food-guide-aliment/basics-base/quantit-eng.php) or call 1-866-225-0709 to get a copy and assess your intake against the suggested daily servings for each of the food groups for women over 50: vegetables and fruit seven; grain products six; milk and alternatives three; and meat and alternatives two. As a result of a compelling seminar at my daughter's school, she quickly learned—at the age of eight—her serving requirements in each of the four food groups and I often hear her chant five, four, two, and one!

I Is for Isoflavones

By mimicking human estrogen at certain sites in the body, isoflavones provide many health benefits that help you to avoid disease. The soybean is loaded with high-quality protein and chock full of vitamins and minerals. Research has linked the consumption of soy products with many health benefits, including protection against breast cancer, prostate cancer, menopausal symptoms, heart disease, and osteoporosis. Many of the health benefits of soy are derived from its isoflavones. Isoflavones are found in soybeans, chickpeas and other legumes. Soybeans are unique because they have the highest concentration of these powerful compounds. There is no RDA for isoflavones from Health Canada but nutritionist Leslie Beck suggests women aim for a daily intake of 60 to 90 milligrams (mg). E.g., ¼ cup of roasted soy nuts has 83 mg. (Sadly, soy sauce has none.) Although the jury is still out on isoflavones, most health professionals recommend eating soy foods for the potential health benefit.

J Is for Junk Food & Processed Foods

A shocking 70% of the foods we eat today are processed in comparison to a mere 10% in the 1950s. When we repeatedly consume processed, fast, convenient foods in lieu of the more nutritional salads, vegetables, fruits and whole grains, we expose our bodies to too many acid-forming foods that can lead to weak bones, poor tooth enamel, and heart disease. This does not mean you have to banish all junk food from your diet. We are all entitled to delve into those desires from time to time. Our family weakness is take-out pizza and potato chips! Bottom line: aim to eat mostly nutritionally and keep the processed food to a minimum.

K Is for Vitamin K

Vitamin K has the potential to be the king of vitamins for bone health. It has received a lot of attention in the last few years for its potential role in osteoporosis. Vitamin K plays a crucial role in blood clotting and, possibly, bone strength and heart health. Vitamin K may help you build stronger bones. More studies are needed, but preliminary research shows that vitamin K activates at least three proteins that appear to play a role in normal bone growth and development. A study from Boston's Tufts University—which has an entire lab devoted to vitamin K research—found that women who ate the least amount of vitamin K-rich foods were more likely to have weaker bones. And in the Harvard Nurses' Health Study involving more than 72,000 women, the risk of hip fracture was 30% lower in women with higher intakes of vitamin K, most of which came from green, leafy vegetables.

Health Canada suggests the adequate daily intake for women is 90 micrograms (ug). A small, one cup spinach salad contains 145 ug. If you eat plenty of fruits and vegetables it is easy to boost your vitamin K intake to 100 micrograms—just one portion of broccoli, cauliflower, or spinach contains more than that amount. Other good sources include: soy products, strawberries, some vegetable oils (soybean, canola, and olive), and liver.

Bottom line: vitamin K may be beneficial in treating osteoporosis but has not been shown to be superior to calcium and vitamin D. It could be promising but it is still too early to recommend vitamin K supplements to reduce the risk of osteoporosis.

L Is for Lycopene

Lycopene is the most potent antioxidant naturally present in many fruits and vegetables and is thought to have cancer fighting abilities. Some findings reveal that lycopene helps reduce bone turnover. St. Michael's University in Ontario is currently studying the role of lycopene in postmenopausal women who are at risk of osteoporosis.

Although it is too early to suggest that eating tomatoes will prevent osteoporosis, it sounds like a good idea to include lycopene in your diet. Leslie Beck suggests a daily intake of 5 to 7 mg. A great way to get your lycopene boost is through a glass of low-sodium tomato juice or through cooked tomatoes (as in tomato sauce) as it is much more available to the body than in raw tomatoes. 1 cup of cooked tomatoes is 9.25 mg versus 1 raw tomato with .8 to 3.8 mg.

M Is for Magnesium

Magnesium is the fourth most abundant mineral in the body and is essential to good health. Approximately 50% of total body magnesium is found in bone. Magnesium is needed for hundreds of biochemical reactions in the body. It helps maintain normal muscle and nerve function, keeps heart rhythm steady, supports a healthy immune system, keeps teeth and bones strong, and helps prevent migraines. Magnesium also helps regulate blood sugar levels and promotes normal blood pressure.

Green vegetables such as spinach are good sources of magnesium because the center of the chlorophyll molecule (which gives green vegetables their colour) contains magnesium. Some legumes (beans and peas), nuts and seeds, and whole, unrefined grains are also good sources of magnesium. Bread made from whole grain wheat flour provides more magnesium than bread made from white refined flour. Eating a wide variety of legumes, nuts, whole grains, and vegetables will help you meet your daily dietary need for magnesium. The RDA is 320 mg. 2 tbsp of wheat bran contains 46 mg.

Bottom line: Leslie Beck sums up some important information on magnesium supplements: "I'd like to clear up one piece of misinformation–magnesium does *not* help your body absorb calcium! Without magnesium, you absorb calcium just fine, but you don't form healthy bones. The mineral helps make parathyroid hormone (PTH), an important regulator of bone-building."

N Is for Niacin

Niacin, also known as vitamin B3, assists in the functioning of the digestive system, skin, and nerves. It is also important for the conversion of food to energy. It is found in dairy products, poultry, fish, lean meats, nuts, and eggs. Legumes and enriched breads and cereals also supply some niacin. The RDA is 14 mg. Vector cereal has 29% of the RDA or about 4 mg.

O Is for Omega-3-6 & 9

Omega fatty acids are polyunsaturated fats. They are healthier than saturated fats and have many functions. Omega-3 and omega-6 fatty acids are essential fatty acids (EFAs). Our bodies cannot manufacture them, and we must consume them in our diets. Omega 9 fatty acids are not essential. Our bodies need omega 9 fats, but we can manufacture them from other sources.

What do EFAs do? They are used by almost every body system, and play a critical role in cellular function. The essential fatty acids support and nourish the brain and nervous system, the heart and circulatory system, and the immune system. They are necessary for healthy skin, hair, and nails.

Health Canada recommends eating fatty fish twice a week, which works out to about 0.5 grams of DHA and EPA a day. The best sources of omega-3 are cold-water fish such as salmon and trout. Other good sources include flaxseed oil and Omega-3 eggs. Omega-6 fatty acids can be found in leafy vegetables, seeds, nuts, grains and vegetable oils (i.e., safflower, sesame, and sunflower). Most diets provide adequate amounts of omega-6. Unless you eat a diet that is extremely low in fat, it is very easy to get more than enough omega-6.

The North American diet is frequently deficient in omega 3 fatty acids. A healthy diet requires a balance of all the essential fatty acids. Include rich sources of omega 3 fatty acid in particular on a regular basis, but make sure you are eating healthy sources of all the EFAs. Keep in mind that whole natural foods are always better sources, as processed foods, such as altered oils, contain less omega fatty acids, if any at all.

There is no RDA for omega but because of their benefits it certainly makes sense to boost your intake. Leslie Beck has four tips to achieve a better balance of omega-6 oils to omega-3 oils:

- Choose lean meats (i.e., extra-lean ground beef) and 1% or skim milk
- Avoid foods with trans fat (i.e., French fries and fast foods) and use margarine with non-hydrogenated fat
- Add one to two tablespoons of flaxseed to your daily diet
- Eat fish at least three times per week. *Canada's Food Guide* recommends at least two.

P Is for Protein

When it comes to bone nutrition, the situation with protein is somewhat of a paradox. While some protein is essential, too much is detrimental. Protein helps the body absorb calcium, and protein is a major building block for bone. By weight, roughly one-third to one-half of our bone is living protein matrix. Protein malnutrition debilitates bone, and can be a significant problem among the elderly in Western countries. Thus, we need to eat protein every day to ensure healthy functioning of our body's immune system; adequate production of hormones and enzymes; and optimal repair and development of muscle, bone, and other body tissues.

Getting the right amount of protein and eating colourful produce daily can lead to bone-building. Too little or too much protein can lead to bone breakdown.

Over-consumption of dietary protein (think of the Atkins and South Beach diets), if not adequately balanced with alkalizing compounds of minerals like calcium, magnesium, and potassium, can lead to bone loss. In this case the loss results from an increased acid load which our bodies must buffer daily by drawing calcium and other alkalizing mineral compounds from the bones.

While adequate protein intake is certainly necessary, the average person in North America consumes far too much protein. If you are a protein lover you just need to remember to balance it with plenty of alkalizing fruits and vegetables. Excess animal protein causes calcium to be excreted by the kidneys.

Not long ago, only animal sources of protein were considered complete and valuable. We were encouraged to eat meat, eggs, and dairy products at virtually every meal. Today nutritional scientists recognize the value of vegetable source proteins from soy foods, legumes (peas, beans, and lentils), nuts, and seeds. Two or more veg- etable-source proteins in combination can provide all the essential amino acids and represent a complete protein. Try these sources to help measure up: grains, legumes, nuts, seeds, and vegetables.

The RDA is .8 grams per kg body weight. For example, if you are 135 pounds (61kg) you need 49 grams of protein each day (61kg X 0.8). 3 oz of chicken has 21 g of protein. This calculation may not work for people who are very overweight or underweight. Check with your doctor and nutritionist to make sure you are eating the amount of protein that is best for your health.

Q Is for Quercetin

Quercetin, found in red apples and other sources, is a type of plant-based chemical known as a flavonoid. In addition to giving plants and flowers their colour, flavonoids do the double duty of serving up a number of health benefits. Quercetin, a powerful antioxidant, has been promoted as being effective against a wide variety of diseases including cancer, especially colon cancer. While some early laboratory results appear promising, as of yet there is no reliable clinical evidence that quercetin can prevent or treat cancer in humans. Quercetin is said to have a number of uses, but most of these are based on early findings from laboratory studies. Some early studies have suggested quercetin helps stimulate osteoblasts and increase bone formation.

The reddish hues found in many plants, vegetables and fruits are the result of quercetin. The pigment is found in red apples, red onions, raspberries, cherries, blueberries, and even red wine. Other sources include grapes, oranges, and other citrus fruits. The dark pigmentation is sometimes absent once the foodstuff is processed but quercetin will still be present, such as in olive oil.

While there is not a recommended dietary allowance (RDA) for quercetin, studies have indicated that toxicity with quercitin is largely a non-issue. However, a dosage of somewhere between 50 mgs and 150 mgs per day is a reasonable dose, and using mega-doses is not recommended. Foods rich in quercetin include black and green tea (2000-2500mg/kg), capers (1800 mg/kg), red apples (44 mg/kg), onion, especially red onion, red grapes, citrus fruit, tomato, broccoli, and other leafy green vegetables, and a number of berries including cherry, raspberry, and cranberry (cultivated 83 mg/kg, wild 121 mg/kg).

R Is for Riboflavin

Help, my urine is bright yellow! No need to be alarmed, it is most likely a result of a multi-vitamin containing riboflavin. When a person's urine becomes bright yellow following high-level supplementation with B-complex vitamins, excess riboflavin excreted in the urine is often responsible for this change in colour. Riboflavin, known as vitamin B2, is an easily absorbed nutrient with a key role in maintaining our health. Like the other B vitamins, B2 plays a key role in energy metabolism and for the metabolism of fats, carbohydrates, and proteins. Also, vitamin B2 is important for body growth, reproduction and red cell production. It has also been shown to help prevent migraines. Milk, cheese, eggs, leafy vegetables, liver, kidneys, legumes, tomatoes, yeasts, mushrooms and almonds are good sources of vitamin B2.

Riboflavin is yellow or yellow-orange in colour and in addition to being used as a food colouring it is also used to fortify some foods. It is used in breakfast cereals, pastas, sauces, fruit drinks, vitamin-enriched milk products, and some energy drinks.

The RDA is 1.1 mg per day. Excellent sources of vitamin B2 include mushrooms (5 oz is about .70 mg), calf liver (4 oz is 2.0 mg) and spinach (1 cup is .40 mg). Very good sources include romaine lettuce (2 cups is .11 mg), asparagus, broccoli, chicken, eggs, yogurt, and milk (1 cup is .40 mg).

S Is for Salt

Sodium is needed in the body to regulate fluids and blood pressure, and to keep muscles and nerves running smoothly—but in very small amounts. Salt used to be hard to come by (which is why ancient Roman soldiers received part of their pay in salt). Now it is readily available and, because our bodies don't have a good mechanism to deal with too much salt, the amount that most North Americans consume is harmful. Too much salt may lead to high blood pressure, a major risk factor for stroke, heart disease, and kidney disease. Eating too much sodium is bad for your bones and can cause bone loss. Like caffeine, sodium also causes the kidneys to excrete calcium. For every 500 mg increase in sodium intake, you must eat an additional 40 mg of calcium to make up for the increased loss.

Salt is sneaky. Almost 80% of dietary sodium North Americans consume comes from processed foods, as opposed to 10% from salt we add at the table and the balance from natural sources from foods. Not surprisingly, the biggest culprits are fast foods. The top ten sources of sodium are: fast food (pizza, submarines, hamburgers and hot dogs), soups, pasta, milk, poultry, potatoes, cheese, cereals (yes cereals!), beef, and sauces.

The RDA for most adults is 1,500 mg per day. North American adults average more than double that amount—3000 mg of sodium daily, considerably higher than the upper limit of 2300 mg (about 1 tsp). One slice of pizza has 1770 mg of salt.

Because I do not like salt on my food, I keep my salt shaker tucked away for when we have guests. So I thought I had a pretty low sodium diet and was easily within the daily intake of 1500 mg of salt. Wrong! Without even reaching for the shaker I consumed more than 2500 mg of sodium. It was hidden in my food choices— in my cereal, hummus, deli meats, hot chocolate, store bought organic soup, milk, etc. The reality is there is plenty of salt hiding in most foods we routinely eat.

I am not suggesting you dissect every meal but I do recommend reading the nutrition labels for sodium content. A cup of Raisin Bran has 40 mg versus Shredded Wheat's 0 mg of sodium. I was surprised to learn that a cup of milk has 115 mg.

Tips to Pass on the Salt:

- Read the Nutrition Facts label and check the sodium content. Try to avoid high sodium products with over 400 mg sodium per serving. Go easy on those with a medium sodium content of 200 to 400 mg per serving. Look for those products that are less than 200 mg per serving.

- Remember that an adequate intake of 1,500 mg of sodium per day implies around 500 mg per meal.

- At the table don't salt your food! Minimize the use of salt in cooking. Sea salt contains almost as much sodium as table salt.

- Try adding a twist of lemon juice, herbs and spices like garlic, curry or ginger, or sodium-free seasonings as an alternative to salt to give flavour a boost. Allow your taste buds to get used to enjoying the subtle flavours of food with less salt. Just as with giving up sugar in coffee, it only takes a short time for your taste to adjust.

- Take the time to read the nutrition information on the websites of your favourite fast food restaurants. Make a note of items with the best nutritional profile.
- Cut down or out processed and packaged foods.

T Is for Tea

Read the tea leaves, caffeine lovers. Tea is gaining ground over coffee. Even popular coffee houses have terrific teas on the menu. The health benefits of tea are one compelling reason. Today, scientific research in both Asia and the West is providing hard evidence for the health benefits long associated with drinking green tea. Preliminary studies show that both green tea and black tea can help reduce cholesterol and prevent heart disease, stroke, and some cancers. Research in Tokyo and Australia suggests that drinking green tea may promote healthy bones and teeth.

A big advantage to tea as a hydration choice lies in the fact that it is a completely natural product, without any added flavorings, colours or preservatives. Likewise, when drunk without adding any sugar, honey, or milk, tea has no calories and simultaneously serves as a crucial component for maintaining the balance of body liquids.

U Is Understanding Canada's Food Labels.

The Nutrition Facts table is found somewhere on all packaged foods in Canada. Take the time to use this great tool to improve your daily diet. It lists calories and 13 nutrients: fat, saturated fat, trans fat, cholesterol, sodium, carbohydrate, fibre, sugars, protein, vitamin A, vitamin C, calcium, and iron.

The first thing you should do when you read the Nutrition Facts is to look at the specific amount of food listed and compare it to how much you actually eat. You can use the Nutrition Facts to compare products more easily, determine the nutritional value of foods, increase or decrease your intake of a particular nutrient after reading this chapter, and assess your diet.

In addition to listing the Percentage Daily Value, the Nutrition Facts table also lists the actual amounts of some nutrients in grams or milligrams. People with specific dietary needs may need to use these values. The Percentage Daily Value is best used as a comparative benchmark when deciding between two food products i.e., if you see 10% daily value for vitamin C in a label on a cereal box that is the percentage of the RDA contained in that specific serving.

All the ingredients in an item are listed in descending order by weight.

Figure 16.1: Nutrition Label Example

Nutrition Facts		
Per 3/4 cup (100 g)		
Amount		% Daily Value
Calories 80		
Fat 1 g		1 %
Saturated Fat 9 g		
Trans Fat 0 g		0 %
Cholesterol 0 mg		
Sodium 2 mg		0 %
Carbohydrate 15 g		5 %
Fiber 3 g		12 %
Sugars 7 g		
Protein 3 g		
Vitamin A	1 %	Vitamin C	2%
Calcium	1 %	Iron	3%

All the nutrient information is based on this amount of food, so compare this with the amount you eat per serving

The **specific amount** is:
- listed under the Nutrition Facts title

- listed in common measures you use at home **and** a metric unit

- not necessarily a suggested quantity of food to consume

www.hc-sc.gc.ca/fn-an/label-etiquet/nutrition/educat/info-nutri-label-etiquet-eng.php

See Interactive nutrition labeling and quiz at:
www.hc-sc.gc.ca/fn-an/label-etiquet/nutrition/cons/interactive-eng.php

V Is for Veggies

The nutrients and minerals required to boost your overall bone and body health come from a wide variety of vegetables. Here are some sneaky ways that I slip these super foods into my family's daily diet: pre-cut carrots and other veggies into small portions that are easily accessible in the fridge; create a salad bar of fruits and veggies for all to choose from at mealtime; toss lots of shredded veggies into dinner dishes such as chili, hamburgers, spaghetti and use less meat; add a variety to sandwiches; and be creative and try veggies you have never had before that are easy to prepare such as spaghetti squash.

If time is a real problem for you, choose frozen vegetables instead of canned vegetables. Frozen vegetables have far less sodium and retain a lot more valuable nutrients.

W Is for Water

Why is water so important? Water, the body's most important nutrient, is involved in every bodily function and makes up 70% of total body weight. Even our solid bones are about 20% water.

We need water to cool our bodies (when we sweat), digest food, carry nutrients and remove waste, cushion organs and joints, and maintain fluid and electrolyte balance. Every day, the body loses about a litre (about 4 cups) of water through normal activity. Exercise uses up even more water. Because, unlike camels, our bodies don't store water, we need to keep drinking it or we risk running dry. It's especially important to keep up your water level while exercising. Drink a glass of water before you work out, stop once or twice during your workout for a drink, and be sure to drink a glass of water after your last exercise. Water helps get rid of excess heat and carries oxygen and nutrients throughout the body, so drinking water prevents early muscle fatigue and helps keep energy up during a long workout.

You can easily get about 20% of your daily fluid need from the foods you eat. Fruits such as watermelon, grapes, oranges, and apples have a high water content. Vegetables like carrots, celery, cucumbers, peppers, lettuce, and tomatoes are also high in water. The other 80% of fluid you need comes from the beverages you drink. Plain water is the best choice. Healthy water sources include tap water, filtered water, milk or juice (fruit or vegetable), or tea (green or black).

Health Canada recommends women drink two to three litres (8 to 12 cups) of water each day. And if you exercise, add another litre (4 cups). Aim to drink 500 milliliters (2 cups) with each meal and your mid-day snack. This is one habit I find very challenging. Although I drink water throughout the day I don't drink half of the required amount! Guilty! While preparing this chapter I have learned some great tips that are helping me increase my intake.

Tips to Ensure You Get Enough Water:

- Carry your personal water bottle for a refreshing drink anytime, anywhere when you are working, traveling, or exercising.

- Keep a glass or cup of water next to you whenever you'll be sitting down for a long time, such as when you're at your desk at work. Drink from it regularly as you're working.

- If you get bored (as I do) with plain water, add a bit of lemon or lime for a touch of flavour.

- Eat water-rich foods, such as fruits like watermelon which is 92% water by weight. A tomato is 95% water.

- Eat vegetables and fruit throughout the day.

- Include additional fluids before, during, and after physical work or play.

- If you drink alcohol, you should drink at least an equal amount of water.

- When you are traveling on an airplane, it is good to drink eight ounces of water for every hour you are on board the plane.

Every day, you lose water through your skin, kidneys, lungs and digestive tract. To keep your body working well, lost water must be replaced. I learned first hand of the consequences of dehydration and the importance of water and fluids. My daughter, at the age of seven, attended a summer outdoor nature camp in sweltering heat. She had a water bottle with her, but we later learned that she had clearly not drank enough. Arriving home one day after camp, she was lethargic, very irritable, and unable to eat or drink. She also had bad stomach cramps that grew more intense. We headed to emergency at the Children's Hospital of Eastern Ontario (CHEO) and quickly received a diagnosis—dehydration. She was treated with a saline IV solution to get rehydrated. This was a lesson learned for all of my family to drink more fluids, especially water.

X Is for Antioxidant

Antioxidants to the rescue! Antioxidants are substances or nutrients in our foods which can prevent or slow the oxidative damage to our body. When our body uses oxygen, it naturally produces free radicals (byproducts of cell activities) which can cause damage. Antioxidants act as "free radical scavengers" and prevent and repair damage done by these free radicals. Oxidative damage contributes to health problems such as heart disease, macular degeneration, diabetes, cancer, and osteoporosis. The more commonly known antioxidants are bright-coloured fruits and vegetables such as carrots, tomatoes, and strawberries. Another rich source is red wine!

Y Is for Yogurt

Not a milk drinker? Reach for yogurt with probiotics. A cup of yogurt has at least as much calcium as an eight-ounce cup of milk. Even if you are lactose intolerant you may be able to eat yogurt with probiotics. There has been a significant buzz in the media making a strong case that everyone needs to add probiotics into their diets for good health. Probiotics means "to promote life" which explains why these nutrients are so important. Probiotics are live microorganisms (in most cases, bacteria) that are similar to beneficial microorganisms found in the human gut. They are also called "friendly bacteria" or "good bacteria."

New research is establishing how important probiotics can be for a variety of conditions. Yogurt containing probiotics may help colon health, boost immunity, lower cholesterol, aid healing after intestinal infections and, as a chaser for antibiotics, yogurt can decrease yeast infections. Yogurt is a rich source of calcium and protein. Examples include Activia from Danone and Yoptimal by Yoplait.

Z Is for Zinc

When people think of vitamins and minerals, most focus on whether they're getting enough A, B, C or D. Too bad. Because zinc is too important to wait until you work through the alphabet to consider it.

Zinc plays a role in the formation of collagen tissue and encourages bone fractures and wounds to heal. Zinc is part of the structure of bones and is necessary for bones to rebuild. Zinc is an essential mineral that is naturally present in some foods, added to others, and available as a dietary supplement. Zinc is also found in many cold lozenges and some over-the-counter drugs sold as cold remedies.

Zinc, a well-known immune system booster, is critical to optimal growth and development. This essential mineral is found in almost every cell, stimulates approximately 100 enzymes and plays a role in everything from taste, brain function and smell acuity to immune system support and DNA synthesis. It also protects the liver from chemical damage and is essential for bone formation. Finally, zinc is vital for maintaining the proper concentration of vitamin E (a factor in blood clotting and healing) in the blood.

Zinc, in minute amounts, is essential for life. Luckily is it found in most types of food. The best sources of zinc are oysters (richest source), red meats, poultry, cheese (ricotta, Swiss, Gouda), shrimp, crab, and other shellfish. Other good, though less easily absorbed, sources of zinc include legumes, whole grains, miso, tofu, brewer's yeast, cooked greens, mushrooms, green beans, tahini, pumpkin, and sunflower seeds.

The RDA is 8 mg/day and the upper limit is 40 mg/day. My name brand multi-vitamin has 15 mg. A cup of milk has .8mg.

The bottom line: before taking supplemental zinc, make sure your needs are not already being met by dietary sources. Moderation with this mineral is a must. Large doses can interfere with the body's ability to absorb other minerals and impair absorption of certain medications. But if you are a vegetarian, over 60, or suspect you're consuming inadequate zinc for any other reason, don't make zinc an afterthought.

Super Foods

Before you reach for supplements to boost your intake of vitamins and minerals try these super foods (recommended by my life wellness coach):

1. All berries (blueberries, raspberries, strawberries, etc.).
2. Dark leafy vegetables (broccoli, spinach, parsley, coriander, bok choy, wild greens).
3. Colourful fruit and vegetables (sweet peppers, tomatoes, carrots, mangoes, oranges, melons, red and purple grapes, plums, cherries, and avocado).
4. Olive oil and flax seed oil (in lieu of other oils).
5. Almonds and walnuts.
6. Salmon and other fatty fish (sardines, mackerel, tuna).
7. Beans and lentils.
8. Oats and oat bran.
9. Yogurt (with probiotics, aka live culture).
10. Water and green tea.

Supplements

The best way to get the daily requirement of essential vitamins is to eat a balanced diet that contains a variety of foods. Specific recommendations depend on age, gender, and other factors such as your bone health.

Vitamin/mineral pills are not insurance for a poor diet! Only food provides you with great taste and the energy you need to get moving and feel great. Some individuals can benefit from supplements such as calcium and vitamin D. Before taking any supplements ask your health care provider which supplements are best for you and talk to a registered dietitian and your pharmacist.

A recent survey shows that 70% of Canadians and 30% of Americans regularly take vitamins and minerals, herbal products, homeopathic medicines and the like—products that have come to be known as natural health products (NHPs). There are endless advertisements on the internet of pills that promise to cure all. Buyer beware! Your doctor's advice is important as some supplements may interfere or interact with other medication you are taking.

The Licensed Natural Health Products Database (LNHPD) contains product-specific information on those natural health products that have been issued a product license by Health Canada. The issuance of a product license means that the product has been assessed by Health Canada and has been found to be safe, effective, and of high quality under its recommended conditions of use. In Canada you can identify licensed natural health products by looking for the eight-digit Natural Product Number (NPN) or Homeopathic Medicine Number (DIN-HM) designation on the label.

The Grocery Store & Kitchen

Healthy eating begins at the grocery store. Fill your cart with whole grain breads and cereals, fruit and vegetables, milk and yogurt, lean meat, poultry, fish, eggs and alternatives such as dried beans, peas and lentils. Read labels to guide your food choices. Here are some creative ways to boost your nutrition that have worked for my family, including my nine-year-old daughter.

1. Eat at least one dark green and one orange vegetable each day.

2. Throw berries onto cereal, into muffins and pancake batter, or on a salad. Add grated vegetables, such as carrot, zucchini or beets, to muffins and cakes.

3. Whirl up a smoothie using milk or orange juice, yogurt, and fruit in a blender. My daughter loves them!

4. Pack fruit and vegetables to take for snacks or lunch every day. Wash and cut in advance, and carry in small plastic bags or containers. This preparation will help increase the odds that it

will get eaten rather than traveling back home. Add fruits and veggies to lunch and dinner.

5. Use flaxseed oil or do half olive oil, half flaxseed oil, for salad dressing.

6. Use *Eating Well with Canada's Food Guide* to figure out how much food you need for good health. For a copy of *Eating Well with Canada's Food Guide*, visit www.healthcanada.gc.ca/foodguide.

7. If you would like help in planning a healthy diet, you can find a Registered Dietitian at www.dietitians.ca/find or by calling 1-888-901-7776.

8. Don't believe that any one food is a magic bullet for health. Instead, choose a variety of foods to help improve your nutritional health.

9. Try a new recipe, a new food or even a different version of your favourite food.

10. The more colourful the food on your plate, the more likely you have chosen fruits and vegetables and foods from various food groups.

In the first months after a fracture, shopping and preparing food may seem daunting. There are workarounds.

• Most grocery stores deliver—a $5 tip to the delivery person and they can often be persuaded to unpack your bags. Depending where you live, you may even be able to shop online for your groceries and have them delivered

• Friends and family asking what they can do to help? Here's a concrete job that they will love to do—give them your shopping list and then ask them to unpack the groceries and even wash, peel, and cube fruits and vegetables for you. Maybe you can organize a cooking party with a couple of good friends to come over for a couple of hours and prep your week's meals while you visit

• If you have the financial resources, you can hire a personal chef to do your shopping and prepare your week's meals for you. It's not as expensive as you might think.

Eating is one of life's greatest pleasures! Make it one of the tools to help your body back to health after fracture—building muscles, stronger bones, upping energy levels and even giving your brain the materials needed to control pain and improve your mood.

Canadians spend about 70 minutes a day eating, while the French spend about 135 minutes a day—and enjoy better physical health. I think it is worth slowing down to better savour our meals and to take the time to explore some of the nutritional content of our daily meals. Enjoying foods rich in nutrients will boost your bones and your overall physical and mental health.

CHAPTER 17

~

KNOWLEDGE IS POWER: MAKING SENSE OF MEDICATIONS & ALTERNATIVE TREATMENTS

Deciding on a drug can be a daunting task. It is difficult to imagine how they work on our bones as we cannot see or feel our bones getting stronger—nor can we feel them getting weaker. Unfortunately, it is often a fracture and the painful consequences that are the wake-up call.

Soon after the diagnosis of my osteoporosis and fractures my doctor prescribed calcitonin to help relieve the pain. I tried the injection form first and then switched to the nasal spray. As neither provided enough relief for my pain and were not considered first line treatments to help improve my bone health, my endocrinologist recommended a bisphosphonate (BP). I readily began the medication without much thought or research as I knew I had to improve my bone health. The alternative—the high risk of another fracture—terrified me.

My first BP was alendronate which I took for five years and then I switched to risedronate because of the severe heartburn I was experiencing. As this steadily worsened I moved to the daily injection of PTH (Forteo). I am now exploring options with a rheumatologist as to what medication to switch to once the two-year therapy of Forteo is complete. Zoledronic acid will most likely be my next option as I am 51 and at a critical stage in life where I could lose bone because of the decline in estrogen. I continue to keep abreast of new drugs such as Denosumab as well as non-pharmaceutical therapy to complement medications such as vibration therapy.

I have suffered the consequences of fractures, so to me the benefits of medication outweigh the risks. The decision to choose an osteoporosis medication is a personal one that should come as a result of doing your homework and having a candid discussion with your doctor—one that includes how and when you will be monitored on the treatment. Should you choose to halt the treatment you should discuss it with your health care team.

The ideal treatment to me would fulfill the following criteria:

- Protect against bone loss
- Enhance BMD at the spine and hip
- Reduce fracture risk at the spine and hip
- Have minimal short-term side effects
- Be available in an annual or semi-annual dosage
- Be safe over long-term use.

Whew, sounds like a lot to ask for! Until that happy day, those of us who require treatments to manage our osteoporosis must do our homework. We must be a part of the decision-making process with our doctor to choose a medication that we are comfortable with. And remember that we are all unique. With our doctor we must assess our own individual risks and benefits for each option and then choose the treatment best for us.

I wrote this chapter in the throes of menopause—the time when most women begin to experience an increased rate of bone loss. At this critical point losing estrogen could wreak havoc on my vulnerable bones. I know that exercise, calcium, and vitamin D are not enough to strengthen my bones and keep me out of the fracture zone. I require medication. In fact, I may need it for the rest of my life as the risk of suffering another broken bone is too great for me.

I am going to be very candid. No one has all the answers on which medication is best for you. The information in this chapter is an overview of medications currently in use (mostly in Canada) or in latter stages of research, as of 2010. I am doing my best to share information that will help prepare you for an open discussion with your doctor on the medication regime (if any is required) to best improve your bone health.

First, my purpose is to put the benefits and risks of osteoporosis medications into both a scientific and a practical perspective. The information I am sharing comes from the best scientific evidence available, my discussions with health experts in the field who treat patients with osteoporosis, and from my own experience as a patient who has used some of these medications

Second, I will shed some light on alternative therapies that don't require a prescription, such as nutritional supplements and the emerging vibration therapy.

Who Needs Medication?

We know that osteoporosis affects both the structure and strength of our bones. Sometimes exercise and good nutrition are not enough to keep your bones out of the fracture zone. The National Osteoporosis Foundation suggests that postmenopausal women and men age 50 and older presenting with the following should be considered for treatment:

- A hip or vertebral fracture

- T-score ≤ -2.5 at the femoral neck or spine after appropriate evaluation to exclude secondary causes

- Low bone mass (T-score between -1.0 and -2.5 at the femoral neck or spine) and a 10-year probability of a hip fracture ≥ 3% or a 10-year probability of a major osteoporosis-related fracture ≥ 20% based on the US-adapted WHO algorithm.

Osteoporosis Canada provides the following guidelines for who should be considered for treatment:

- Patients at high risk (> 20% probability for major osteoporotic fracture over 10 years)

- Patients with a fragility fracture of the hip or vertebra, or more than one fragility fracture as this constitutes a high risk for future fracture

- Patients at moderate risk (10 to 20% probability for major osteoporotic fracture over 10 years) may undergo other tests such as an x-ray to determine if they have a vertebral fracture prior to deciding if medication would be beneficial.

For those at moderate fracture risk, patient preference and other risk factors should be used to guide the decision as to whether medication would be beneficial.

Goal of Medication

The job of the osteoporosis medication is to decrease your risk of fracture. The best measure of success? No new fractures after taking the medication faithfully for 6 to 12 months.

There is no known cure for osteoporosis. Fortunately, there are steps you can take to prevent, slow, or stop its progress by improving bone density and in some cases reverse the disorder to some degree. Medications can help maintain or improve the bone health of most people. These medicines do not actually "fix" the problems that cause osteoporosis. Instead, they work by suppressing the activity of the osteoclasts or encouraging the osteoblasts to work harder to build new bone. I compare it to repairing a road—some drugs inhibit osteoclasts—in other words, they stop formation of new potholes and fill in some of the old potholes but they do not apply a new layer of asphalt. Other drugs stimulate the osteoblasts to form more bone, meaning a true new layer of asphalt.

The most important factor that doctors consider when prescribing drugs for osteoporosis is how it will reduce your risk of fracture. This is accomplished by slowing or stopping bone loss and maintaining or increasing bone strength. Osteoporosis drugs work by improving the quality of your bones as well as the density of your bones. Bone strength depends on both bone quality and bone mineral density (BMD). Changes in BMD alone may not always reflect fracture risk.

Osteoporosis drugs work on improving the quality of your bones, and that can't be measured with an increase in bone density. There are substances that can be measured in the blood or urine (bone markers) that can indicate how rapidly osteoclasts are breaking down bone and how effectively osteoblasts are at restoring new bone. To date, bone markers have been very useful for research to determine the onset of drug action but they are not yet routinely used for diagnosis and management of osteoporosis. Doctors may choose to review bone markers to help:

- Diagnose osteoporosis

- Identify "fast bone losers" and patients at high risk of fracture

- Select the best treatment for osteoporosis

- Provide an early indication of the response to treatment.

Bone is lost slowly over years and it requires considerable time to regain bone. Patience is vital, as it can take years of therapies before bone density improves. The good news is that fracture risk reductions from therapy occur much more rapidly than BMD changes—sometimes within weeks of starting treatment. Many researchers believe that the quick improvement in fracture risk is due to microscopic changes in the structure of the bones that make them stronger and less likely to break. These microscopic changes happen in addition to the improvement of the total bone present. Presumably, treatment strengthens the bone through changes independent of BMD, such as a decrease in bone remodeling rate.

Your doctor will recommend BMD testing to see if your medication is keeping your bone density stable. The frequency of testing (from 1 to 5 years apart) depends on your doctor, your present bone health, your risk of fracture and provincial/territorial or state guidelines for BMD.

The Evidence that Medication Helps Bones

The number of studies on osteoporosis medications is over-whelming! Some of us enjoy delving into studies on osteoporosis. It empowered me—the more I understood and knew, the more comfortable I felt as an equal partner with my doctors and other health care professionals. Others may find it overwhelming and too draining. If you do want to review some of the studies, it is important to get the background on the clinical trial. Clinical trials are research studies in which people help doctors find ways to improve health.

My research led me to two very significant documents. For each document, a team of experts assessed studies for treatments available and shared the findings from the highest quality studies:

1. The 2002 comprehensive guide released by the Ottawa Health Research Institute titled: *Making Choices: Osteoporosis Treatment Options, A Decision Guide for Women with Osteoporosis Considering Treatment Options to Prevent Further Bone Loss and Fractures.*

2. Management of osteoporosis in menopausal women: 2010 position statement of The North American Menopause Society (NAMS). *Menopause: The Journal of The North American Menopause Society,* Vol. 17, No. 1, pp. 23-56.

Making Sense of Studies

Each study tries to answer scientific questions and to find better ways to prevent, diagnose or treat disease and its side effects. You want to be sure the study:

* Is randomized. This means that people are randomly assigned to two groups—one group receives the drug being tested, the other group receives a placebo or comparator drug. An even stronger study method, the Double Blind, means that the scientists also don't know who is getting the active medications. Randomization is a process that assigns research participants by chance, rather than by choice, to either the investigational group or the control group of the clinical trial. Each study participant has a fair and equal chance of receiving either the new intervention being studied or of receiving the existing or "control" intervention.

  Research participants are randomized in clinical trials so that bias does not weaken the study results. Bias consists of human choices, beliefs or any other factors besides those being studied that can affect a clinical trial's results. If physicians or participants themselves choose the group, assignments might be personally influenced and therefore unevenly slanted toward one side or the other.

  For instance, if a study is not randomized, physicians might unconsciously assign participants with a more hopeful prognosis to the experimental group, making the new therapy seem more effective than it really is. Conversely, participants with a less hopeful prognosis might pick the experimental treatment, leading it to look less effective than it really is

- Concludes with researchers being confident about the results
- Uses an adequate number of people and that most participants completed the study
- Covers a substantial period of time on the medication (i.e., one year or more).

Approved Classes of Osteoporosis Medications

Biotechnology companies continually work on developing new therapies because this disease affects millions of individuals. The currently approved classes of drugs are categorized as:

- Bisphosphonates
- Calcitonin
- Hormone therapy
- Selective estrogen receptor modulators (SERMS)
- Anabolic agents (parathyroid hormone)
- Human monoclonal antibody that prevents RANKL.

When reviewing medication options take a look at how the drug improves BMD, how effective it is at reducing the risk of spinal fractures and hip fractures, and possible side effects.

Keep Taking Your Medication

As many as 50% of women on osteoporosis medication stop treatment after less than one year, putting themselves at risk of fracture.

There are many reasons why we play dice with our bones:

- Fear of unwanted side effects, often emphasized by the media
- Limited knowledge of what the treatment is doing and how long it will take
- Inconvenience—many of us can't manage to take a vitamin pill regularly!

- Cost

- Reluctance to take prescription medications—this is where I had to realize that a true holistic approach uses ALL available resources; medication, meditation, nutrition, exercise, and physiotherapy were all part of my bone health continuum

- Doubts regarding their real effectiveness in reducing the risk of fracture

- Lack of awareness about the risk and consequence of fracture. If you haven't had a fracture, it is almost impossible to imagine how much it will change your life and how hard you will need to work to recover from it.

Every medication comes with the risk of side effects. They can be mild or severe, temporary or permanent. Side effects won't affect each person who takes medication, but the possibility does keep us worrying. I liken it to crossing the street. My decision to cross is based on adding up various risk factors against the benefits. If it's raining heavily during rush hour, it's safer for me to suffer the "side effect" of getting wet for an extra 2 minutes and wait for the light to change and traffic to come to a full stop. On a sunny Sunday, with no cars in either direction, I might choose to jaywalk (as long as my daughter isn't with me). Unfortunately, the difficulty in seeing how our bones are doing means that half of us choose to "jaywalk" with our medication, wrongly perceiving a sunny Sunday when it's actually heavy rain.

Discuss the risks and benefits of medications with your doctor. Many people, including myself, hesitate to include medication in their strategy to manage osteoporosis. If you do your homework and then decide to follow a therapy over the recommended period of time to benefit from it, you will be comfortable with your decision. If doubts remain, chances of abandoning the treatment prematurely are very high.

Questions about Medication Options to Research & Discuss with Your Doctor

- How well does the medication reduce the risk of spine fracture?

- How well does the medication reduce the risk of hip fracture?

- How well does the medication increase BMD?
- Your age, medical history and other medications you are taking in relation to how it affects your treatment options
- Your risk of fracture (i.e., 10 year probability of fracture)
- The purpose of the medication
- What dosing option might work best for you to ensure you continue using the medication?
- Possible side effects. Share and discuss your concerns and doubts with your doctor
- The cost of the medication and whether it is covered by the province/territory or state drug plan or your own insurance plan or if you can afford to pay for it. (See Osteoporosis Drug Coverage in Canada Osteoporosis Update Winter 2010 vol.14 no.1 p.9)
- Contraindications—if you are being treated with medication for another issue, will adding your osteoporosis drug to the mix create problems. Other medications, foods, and even sunlight can make a drug less or more potent, which can cause serious problems
- How and when you will be monitored, BMD tests, blood work, etc.

Most of the medications described in this chapter are proven to increase bone density and lower the risk of a spinal fracture. Some have proven to lower the risk of fractures of the spine and the hip. Many of the studies on the effectiveness of these medications have been done on postmenopausal women.

The important information I wanted to know when I began investigating medication options was:

- What each drug is
- How it works on the bones
- Its effect on BMD and reducing risk of fracture
- Forms (pill, IV, liquid, etc.) and dosing options

- Possible side effects and other things to consider about the medication.

For commercial reasons, the same medication might be sold under a different name in different countries. I live in Canada, so I've used the Canadian brand-names—you can check online or ask your doctor if it goes by a different name.

What is the Best Treatment for Osteoporosis in Postmenopausal Women?

(the information below was obtained from Osteoporosis Canada *2010 Clinical Practice Guidelines*. See www.osteoporosis.ca for up-to-date information.)

Table 17. 1

Type of fracture	Antiresorptive Therapy						Bone Formation Therapy
	Bisphosphonates			Denosumab	Raloxifene	Estrogen ** (Hormone Therapy)	Teripara-tide
	Alendronate	Risedronate	Zoledronic acid				
Vertebral	√	√	√	√	√	√	√
Hip	√	√	√	√	-	√	-
Non-vertebral***	√	√	√	√	-	√	√

First Line Therapies with Evidence for Fracture Prevention in Postmenopausal Women*

* For postmenopausal women, √ indicates first line therapies and Grade A recommendation

** Hormone therapy (estrogen) can be used as first-line therapy in women with post menopausal symptoms

*** In Clinical trials, non-vertebral fractures are a composite endpoint including hip, femur, pelvis, tibia, humerus, radius, and clavicle.

Note: According to OC, calcitonin or etidronate can be considered for prevention of vertebral fractures among those intolerant of first-line therapies.

Antiresorptive & Anabolic Agents

Medications fall into two categories: antiresorptive agents and anabolic agents. Calcitonin, bisphosphonates, hormone therapy, selective estrogen receptor modulators (SERMS) and denosumab are medications that slow down bone loss by inhibiting the development and activation of osteoclasts (the cells that eat way at bone). When you start these medications, you stop losing bone as quickly as before. The goal of treatment with these antiresorptive medications is to prevent bone loss and lower the risk of breaking bones.

Teriparatide, a form of parathyroid hormone, is the first osteoporosis medication to increase the rate of bone formation in the bone remodeling cycle and is in a distinct category of osteoporosis medications called **anabolic drugs**. This is currently the only osteoporosis medication in Canada that rebuilds bone. The goal of treatment with teriparatide is to build bone and lower the risk of breaking bones.

Antiresorptive Medications
Calcitonin

What is Calcitonin?

Calcitonin is a naturally occurring hormone made by the human thyroid gland and certain glands in fish and birds. It helps regulate the calcium levels in the body.

How does Calcitonin work on the bones?

Scientists found that both synthetic and natural calcitonin slow down the osteoclasts that break down bone which allows the bone-building osteoblasts to work more effectively. The calcitonin given in therapy is similar to that found in salmon because the fish form is close to human calcitonin but is more potent.

Calcitonin can maintain or increase bone mass in the spine, and decrease the risk of fractures to the spine. It can also provide partial relief from bone pain, especially acute pain from a spinal fracture, for some people.

How well does Calcitonin work on the bones?

In postmenopausal women, Calcitonin was found to:
- Increase bone density by 1 to 3% over two years

- Reduce the risk of spine fracture by 31%
- Have no major effect on reducing hip fracture risk.

Things to consider about Calcitonin
Calcitonin is not as effective as other medications described in this chapter to treat osteoporosis.

What forms does Calcitonin come in?
Calcitonin is not effective as a pill as it is broken down during digestion. Calcitonin nasal spray (brand name Miacalcin) is approved for the treatment of osteoporosis in women who have been post-menopausal for at least five years. Calcitonin injection (brand name Calcimar Solution, Caltine) is currently not approved for the treatment of osteoporosis but is sometimes prescribed for people who have fractures of the vertebrae, mainly to relieve pain.

Possible side effects of Calcitonin:
- Flushing (feeling of warmth) of the face or hands

- Nausea

- Nasal irritation (nasal spray)

- Injection site reactions (injectable form).

Table 17.2: Summary of Calcitonin

Medication and Brand Names	Pros	Cons
Calcitonin (Miacalcin-nasal spray, Calcimar Solution, Caltine-injectable form)	Modest increase in BMD in the spine; pain relief for spine fractures; reduces risk of spine fractures	No effect on hip BMD or hip fracture risk

Bisphosphonates

What are they?
Bisphosphonates (BPs) reduce fracture risk at the hip and spine. This is why they are the most widely prescribed treatment for those

with, or at risk for, osteoporosis. They are a class of non-hormonal drugs that have been used since the 1960's to treat various bone disorders.

With osteoporosis, the cells that take bone away *(osteoclasts)* work faster than the cells that build bone *(osteoblasts)*. BP molecules "stick" to calcium and to the material bone is made of and bind to them. BPs stop the osteoclasts from removing bone. Overall, the major way that BPs improve bone strength is that they prevent perforations in the bone that weaken the structure of the bone.

The evolution of BPs has led to compounds with ever-increasing potency in terms of suppressing the osteoclasts. Second-generation drugs like alendronate are up to 100 times more potent than first-generation compounds like etidronate. Third-generation drugs are even stronger, with zoledronic acid more potent than all other BPs.

When BPs are taken orally only a small amount enters the blood and gets to the bone—most of it passes through the kidneys. When the drug is given by intravenous infusion, about half of it goes into the bone.

Etidronate/calcium (brand name Didrocal)

This contains two different medications, etidronate and calcium carbonate, to be taken at different times.

Etidronate is an effective inhibitor of bone resorption. It is not suitable for continuous dosing because it interferes with the mineralization of newly forming bone and may cause softening of the bones (osteomalacia). If you and your doctor decide that is the right medication option, you will take etidronate for 14 days and then calcium supplements for 76 days. You may then repeat this cycle.

In the US, etidronate is approved only for the treatment of Paget's disease (weakened and deformed bones) but not for osteoporosis therapy.

How well does etidronate work on the bones?
Etidronate is not as effective as other BPs, but it can be an option for women unable to tolerate other medications. Studies show that:

- it increases bone density by 2 to 4% over two years
- it reduces the risk of a spinal fracture by 37%
- there is no apparent reduction in risk of hip fracture.

Possible side effects of etidronate
- Nausea and diarrhea
- Headache and dizziness
- Abdominal pain.

Long-term issues
- Softening of the bone (osteomalacia).

Alendronate (brand names Fosamax & Fosavance—alendronate plus vitamin D3)

Fosomax is available in pill form that can be taken once a day or once a week.

Fosavance is available as a weekly pill. This is a combination medication that contains alendronate and vitamin D3 (cholecalciferol), needed for calcium absorption and healthy bones. This may be suggested to women with osteoporosis and low vitamin D levels.

Risedronate (brand name Actonel)

This is available in pill form that can be taken daily, weekly, or monthly.

Actonel with calcium is a combo pack with two different medications, risedronate and calcium. The risedronate is taken on day 1 and then the calcium is taken for the next 6 days. Then the cycle starts again.

How well do alendronate and risedronate work on the bones?
Studies show that Alendronate (Fosomax):

- Increases bone density 4 to 7% over 2 years
- Reduces the risk of spine fracture by 48%
- Reduces the risk of hip fracture by 40%.

Studies show that Risedronate (Actonel):
- Increases bone density 3 to 4% over 2 years

- Reduces the risk of spine fracture by 37%

- Reduces the risk of hip fracture by 39%.

Things to consider
- BP tablets are poorly absorbed so they must be taken first thing in the morning on an empty stomach, with only water

- You must remain upright (sitting, standing, or walking) for 30 minutes

- You must wait 30 minutes (two hours for etidronate) before eating, drinking, or taking any other medications.

Possible side effects of alendronate and risedronate
- Heartburn

- Irritation of the esophagus (tube connecting the throat to the stomach)

- Stomach problems and ulcers

- Headache, nausea and diarrhea

- Pain in the muscles or joints.

Zoledronic acid (brand name Aclasta)

This is given once a year as an intravenous (IV) infusion. It is the only intravenous medication proven effective at reducing the risk of fractures in patients with osteoporosis.

How well does zoledronic acid work on the bones?
Studies show zoledronic acid (Aclasta):
- increases BMD by 6 to 7% over 3 years

- reduces risk of spine fracture by 70%

- reduces risk of hip fracture by 41%.

Things to consider about zoledronic acid
Zoledronic acid is given as a yearly intravenous (IV) dose in a doctor's office or other outpatient setting. Prior to getting their annual

infusion, patients need to have blood tests for creatinine levels (kidney function) and calcium to confirm that the blood calcium level is normal.

Possible side effects of zoledronic acid
- Flu-like symptoms

- Fever, pain in muscles or joints, and a headache. These normally stop within 2-3 days and usually do not happen with future infusions

- The IV must be given slowly (at least 15 minutes) to avoid damage to the kidneys.

Other BP medications that you may have read about:

Pamidronate (brand name Aredia)

Pamidronate is given by intravenous and is used to treat cancer that has spread to bones. It can help suppress osteoclast activity and reduce bone pain. Because there is no evidence of fracture reduction with intravenous pamidronate it is not recommend by Osteoporosis Canada as a treatment for osteoporosis.

Ibandronate (brand name Boniva)

Ibandronate, approved in the US but not in Canada, is available as a daily or monthly pill or by intravenous every three months. (You may have seen the Boniva ads with the actress Sally Field as the spokesperson.) Studies show that it increases BMD and reduces the risk of spinal fractures but that it does not reduce the risk of a hip fracture.

Making Sense of the Media on Side Effects of Bisphosphonates

Fresh disasters sell newspapers and keep us glued to TV and websites. There are rare but very serious conditions that may develop in people using bisphosphonate (BP) medications including:
- Osteonecrosis of the jaw (ONJ) in which the living bone tissue of the jaw is damaged

- Irregular heart rhythm

- Cancer of the esophagus
- Unusual breaks in the thigh bone.

For the estimated 30 million people in North America who take a BP (including me) this is alarming news! Sometimes women increase their risk of fracture by abruptly stopping their treatment. While these conditions are serious, the number of people with them remains tiny compared to the number of people who have taken BPs to treat osteoporosis.

I had a hard look at the statistical chance of developing one of these conditions versus the probability of a future spinal or hip fracture and discussed it with my health care team. It may help to look at it this way—people die in car accidents. But there are millions and millions of car trips for each person who is killed. Each time we get into a car we have unconsciously done a risk assessment, based on our available information, and decided that the benefit outweighed the risk. For me, the solid data that the drugs would reduce my chance of future fracture outweighed the very small risk that I might develop serious complications.

Osteonecrosis of the Jaw (ONJ)

Osteonecrosis (ONJ) is a rare but nasty dental condition when exposed jaw bone shows no sign of healing. ONJ is much more likely to occur after an invasive dental procedure, such as having a tooth pulled or implant surgery.

In general, ONJ is a rare condition. The chances of developing jaw bone damage from using any BP is very small. Of the millions of people who have used BPs over the years, a relatively small number of cases of jaw damage have been reported as of May 2010. Of those cases, the majority are in cancer patients using the intravenous form of a BP. Your risk could increase, however, if you have certain dental procedures such as having a tooth pulled, as the jaw bone becomes exposed. Even though your chances of developing ONJ are rare, it is a good idea to tell your dentist if you are taking a BP.

In early 2005 the FDA in the United States released a statement saying that osteonecrosis is a risk with all forms of bisphosphonate, not just the IV form. The cause of ONJ and BPs is a topic of great debate and the data is highly controversial. The exact nature of the relationship is unknown. Some researchers believe that BPs prevent the formation of new blood vessels within jaw tissue, compromising the natural healing process of the jawbone, leading to death of the tissue and the eventual collapse of the bone.

If you are not currently taking a BP, but will be starting one soon, be sure to tell your dentist now. They may want to take care of necessary dental work and allow the mouth to heal before you start taking your BP. Patients already taking a BP may want to consider (after consultation with their doctors) a drug holiday that starts shortly before dental procedure and lasts until the gums and jaw have healed—although there is as yet no clinical evidence that this makes a difference in ONJ.

Report Symptoms

If you have been treated with a BP and have side effects or unusual symptoms be sure to report these to your doctor and dentist immediately, especially if they include: pain, swelling, or infection of the gums, loosening of teeth, poor healing of the gums, or numbness or the feeling of heaviness in the jaw.

Osteoporosis Canada Position Statement

June 2007

At present, there is simply not enough medical information to prepare fact-based guidelines for the prevention and treatment of ONJ in patients taking oral BPs for treatment of osteoporosis or Paget's Disease. The risk of developing ONJ with oral BPs is known to be very low: between 1 in 10,000 and 1 in 100,000.

Jan. 2008

Our experts conclude that we need more research in order to see if there is any sort of connection between osteoporosis or the medications we use to treat it and osteonecrosis of bone. What remains clear is that the risk of fracture in those with osteoporosis is high and that BPs can decrease this risk very significantly.

Although there are fewer media reports on concerns of atrial fibrillation, cancer of the esophagus, and unusual fractures in the thigh bone associated with the use of BPs, it is helpful to keep abreast of any updates by checking both the osteoporois.ca and nof.org websites.

Health Canada did issue this advisory on August 9, 2005 regarding zoledronic acid (Aclasta): This medication has been shown to increase the risk of atrial fibrillation (irregular heartbeat) in some clinical trials. Contact your doctor if you feel palpitations, a rapid and irregular heartbeat, dizziness, weakness, or shortness of breath.

My final thought? There is a very faint chance for most osteoporosis patients of developing one of these effects—as scary as they are—and a much greater chance of painful and potentially crippling fracture(s) if you do not use medication to build up bone strength. Be very clear about the odds in each direction before you make a decision.

Do Your Homework

As you can see, any medication comes with a risk of a side effect. If you have concerns regarding your treatment and possible side effects do your homework before going to speak with your doctor and dentist. Look for the updated position statements by the International Osteoporosis Foundation, the US Food and Drug Administration (FDA), Osteoporosis Canada, Health Canada and your province/territory or state's health website.

How Long Should I Take a Bisphosphonate?

There are no evidence-based guidelines or clear medical consensus on how long people with osteoporosis should take BPs. Some research has shown that the process of bone breakdown will rise when the BP is discontinued. Other results suggest that for some women, stopping BP treatment may be possible after five years. However, women at high risk of fracture may benefit by continuing beyond five years.

I found the following statement from the National Osteoporosis Foundation contained a practical suggestion:

March 2010
Reviewing Your Treatment Plan

If you are taking an osteoporosis medicine, it is important that you review your treatment plan every year with your doctor or other healthcare provider. If you have been taking an osteoporosis medicine for five years, discuss the benefits of continuing it.

People who are not at high risk of breaking a bone may be able to take a "drug holiday" after five years of treatment with BPs. This means that you stop taking your osteoporosis medicine (BP) but continue to see your healthcare provider to monitor your bone health, and look forward to restarting it at some point in the future. This does not apply to other medicines given for osteoporosis.

If you are at high risk of breaking a bone, then you may benefit by staying on an osteoporosis medicine. Other people may benefit from switching to a different medicine. Your healthcare provider is the best person to guide you about whether you should start, continue, switch or stop an osteoporosis medicine. Again, it is always important to look at both the benefits and risks of taking a medicine.

Table 17.3: Summary of Bisphosphonates

Brand Names	Pros	Cons
Alendronate (Fosomax) Risedronate (Actonel) Zoledronic acid (Aclasta)	Improves BMD Reduces the risk of fracture in both spine and hip	Gastrointestinal problems, heartburn, joint and muscle pain Very rare: Osteonecrosis of the Jaw (ONJ), atrial fibrillation, cancer of the esophagus, and unusual fractures in the thigh bone.

Hormone Therapy (HT)

Most of us are aware of hormone therapy (HT) as it relates to menopause. It is used to relieve symptoms such as hot flashes, night sweats, and mood swings. HT is not the first choice for osteoporosis prevention but it may prevent bone loss and fractures in women who are using HT for symptom control.

How does Hormone Therapy work on the bone?

In the 1980's hormone therapy was considered the most effective means of protecting against the rapid loss of bone that follows menopause. During the years leading up to our final period (perimenopause) our ovaries become smaller and make less of the hormone estrogen. There is a direct connection between the loss of estrogen and the loss of bone, particularly trabecular bone.

How well does Hormone Therapy work on the bone?

HT increases estrogen levels. This slows down bone loss and may even help increase bone density after an osteoporosis diagnosis.

Studies show that hormone therapy:

- Increases bone density 5 to 7% over 2 years
- Reduces risk of hip fracture by 34%
- Reduces risk of spine fracture by 30%.

Things to consider

The decision to take hormone therapy should not be an impulsive one. It is critical to weigh the benefits and risks and discuss them with your doctor. Many studies have shown that HT is associated with increased risks for certain cancers and cardiovascular events. While the French E3N study—the first to look at hard data over time and with a large number of participants indicates that bioidentical hormones may avoid these risks (Arteriosclerosis, Thrombosis, & Vascular Biol.2010; 30: 340-345)—lack of standardized manufacturing can be an issue. Osteoporosis Canada states that HT (estrogen) can be used as a first-line therapy for women with menopausal symptoms.

Excerpt from the North American Menopause Society Position Statement 2010

The benefit-risk ratio for menopausal HT is favourable for women who initiate HT close to menopause but decreases in older women and with time since menopause in previously untreated women.

An individual risk profile is essential for every woman contemplating any regimen of EPT (estrogen plus progestogen) or ET (estrogen). Women should be informed of known risks, but it cannot be assumed that benefits and risks of HT apply to all age ranges and durations of therapy. A woman's willingness to accept risks of HT will vary depending on her individual situation, particularly whether HT is being considered to treat existing symptoms or to lower risk for osteoporotic fractures that may or may not occur. Moreover, because incidence of disease outcomes increases with age and time since menopause, the benefit-risk ratio for HT is more likely to be acceptable for short-term use for symptom reduction in a younger population. In contrast, long-term HT or HT initiation in older women may have a less acceptable ratio.

Extended use of HT is an option for women who have established reduction in bone mass, regardless of menopause symptoms; for prevention of further bone loss and/or reduction of osteoporotic fracture when alternate therapies are not appropriate or cause side effects; or when the benefits of extended use are expected to exceed the risks. The optimal time to initiate HT and the optimal duration of therapy have not been established, but HT would largely be used in the early years after menopause. The benefits of HT on bone mass dissipate quickly after discontinuation of treatment.

Hormone Therapy form & dosing options

Hormone therapy is estrogen or combination estrogen/ progesterone medication. Estrogen is a female hormone that brings about changes in other organs in the body. It generally comes from animal sources. Progesterone is a female hormone that prepares the uterus for a pregnancy each month. The synthetic form of progesterone is progestin. There are various types and brands of estrogen and progesterone available in a large variety of dosage forms such as tablets, patches, creams, and vaginal rings.

Estrogen and progesterone are usually combined because estrogens taken alone increase the risk for endometrial cancer—the uncontrolled growth and spread of abnormal cells from the inner lining of the uterus. Women without a uterus (i.e., those who have had a hysterectomy) do not need to take progesterone.

Possible side effects

- Increased risk of blood clots, pulmonary embolism, and deep vein thrombosis

- Increases risk of stroke

- Increases risk of heart attack

- Increases risk of breast cancer with long-term use (beyond 4 years)

- Increases ovarian cancer deaths (after 10 years of estrogen)

- Breast tenderness, vaginal spotting.

Table 17.4: Summary of Hormone Therapy

Brand Names	Pros	Cons
There are many different brand names, including Prempro, Premplus, Estracomb	Improves BMD Reduces risk of fracture in the spine and hip	Increased risk of: blood clots, breast cancer, cardiovascular problems, heart attack, stroke

Selective Estrogen Receptor Modulators (SERMs)

Selective Estrogen Receptor Modulators (SERMs) have been developed to provide the beneficial effects of estrogens without their potential disadvantages. They are not hormones. They are a class of drugs that mimic estrogen in some tissues but act to block estrogen's effects in others. That is why they are said to be selective.

How do SERMs work on the bones?

SERMs are designed to do all the good things that estrogen does. They mimic the positive effects of estrogen on bone and block the effects of estrogen on other parts of the body such as the uterus and the breast.

How well do SERMs work on the bones?

Although various newer SERMs are presently being developed, the only SERM approved in Canada for the prevention and treatment of osteoporosis is raloxifene, marketed as Evista.

Studies show raloxifene:

- Increases bone density 2.5% over 2 years
- Reduces risk of spine fracture by 41%
- Has no significant effect on reducing risk of hip fracture.

Forms and dosing options

Raloxifene (Evista) comes as a pill and is taken once a day.

Possible side effects

- Increases risk of blood clots, especially in older women with heart disease (similar to that seen with women using HT)
- Hot flashes
- Leg cramps.

Things to consider

Raloxifene prevents bone loss and reduces risk of spinal fractures but its effectiveness in reducing other fractures is uncertain. The benefits of raloxifene in reducing the risks of a spinal fracture should be weighed against the increased risks of blood clots and a fatal stroke. When considering raloxifene talk to your doctor about the benefits and risks of this option versus other options listed in this chapter.

Table 17.5: Summary of SERMs

Medication and Brand Names	Pros	Cons
SERMs (Raloxifene marketed as Evista)	Modest increase in BMD; reduces risk of spine fracture; reduction in breast cancer and "bad" LDL cholesterol	No effect on hip fracture risk; increase in hot flashes; risk of blood clots

Denosumab (brand name Prolia)

What is Denosumab?

Denosumab, the first drug in its class, is a biologic agent that claims to mimic the body's natural mechanism for blocking the formation of bone-destroying cells.

How does denosumab work on the bones?

Denosumab inhibits bone resorption by the osteoclasts. It is designed to target RANKL (RANK ligand), a protein that acts as the primary signal to promote the formation of new osteoclasts and bone removal by the osteoclasts. In many bone loss conditions, RANKL overwhelms the body's natural defense against bone destruction. In simpler terms, it helps stop the development of bone-removing cells before they cause bone loss.

How well does denosumab work on the bones?

In postmenopausal women with low bone mass, denosumab:

- Increased BMD of the spine by 9% and the hip by 6%

- Reduced the risk of spinal fractures by 68%

- Reduced the risk of hip fracture by 40%

- One study showed that denosumab increased BMD at the forearm, which is mainly cortical bone. This raises the hope that it might better protect bones like the hip that have a large percentage of cortical bone.

Forms of and dosing options

It is given by injection just under the skin, twice yearly, by a trained healthcare professional, so it may be seen to be much more convenient than medications that have to be taken daily or weekly.

Possible side effects

- Urinary, pancreatitis or ear infections

- Pain in the muscles, arms, legs or back

- Skin problems such as infections, eczema and rashes

- Low calcium levels in the blood

- In rare cases osteonecrosis of the jaw (ONJ).

Things to consider

Denosumab was approved by the FDA and Health Canada in 2010 for the treatment of postmenopausal women with osteoporosis at high risk for fracture or patients who have failed or are intolerant to other available osteoporosis therapy.

Do not take Denosumab if you have been told by your doctor that your blood calcium level is too low.

While extensive trial data have demonstrated Denosumab's ability to build bone mineral density and prevent fractures, the therapy is newly approved in Canada. Doctors may recommend other treatments until more long-term safety data becomes available.

Table 17.6: Summary of Denosumab

Medication and Brand Names	Pros	Cons
Denosumab (Prolia)	Significant increase in BMD in the spine and hip; reduces risk of spine and hip fracture	Rare but a concern; low calcium levels in the blood; osteonecrosis of the jaw (ONJ).

Anabolic Agents

Teriparatide (brand name Forteo)

Teriparatide, a man-made form of the hormone parathyroid that exists naturally in the body, is the first treatment that does not simply halt bone loss, but increases bone mass by stimulating new bone formation, reducing the chance of a fracture. (Antiresorptive therapies slow the bone remodeling and resorptive processes, but they have no direct effect on bone formation.)

How does Teriparatide work on the bone?

Teriparatide forms new bone, increases bone mineral density, and bone strength. It stimulates new bone formation by increasing the number and activity of bone forming cells—the osteoblasts. Our bodies naturally produce a hormone called parathyroid that regulates calcium levels in the body. If the calcium levels in the blood drop a little bit, the parathyroid glands kick into gear and make parathyroid hormone (PTH) which stimulates osteoclasts to get calcium from bone during resorption. When the calcium in the blood is at an optimal level, then the parathyroid glands stop making PTH.

I was bewildered when I read that early research found that PTH adjusted calcium by stimulating the osteoclasts to dissolve bone. But more recent research showed that PTH, when not given continuously (i.e., only once a day), also stimulates the bone-growing osteoblasts, which led to the use of PTH to treat osteoporosis.

How well does teriparatide work on the bone?

Studies show that teriparatide:

- Increases BMD by 9% in the spine and 3% in the hip over 2 years
- Reduces risk of spinal fractures by 65%
- Reduces risk of non-vertebral fractures by 53%.

Form and dosing of teriparatide

Teriparatide (brand name Forteo) is self-administered as a daily injection, into the abdomen or thigh from a pre-loaded pen containing a 28 day supply of medication. Whoever is administering the injection (patient or caregiver) is trained in the proper use of the pen by a health care professional. Each pen must be stored in the fridge and can be used up to 28 days.

Teriparatide can be taken for a maximum of two years at which in time, in order to keep the gain in bone benefits, most experts recommend that patients start an antiresorptive medication. Studies show that women who did not receive subsequent treatment with a BP lost BMD over two to three years after stopping teriparatide.

Possible side effects

- dizziness and nausea

- leg cramps

- modest elevations in serum and urine calcium can occur, but there is no documented increase in the risk of kidney stones.

During the drug testing process, studies in rats given 3 to 60 times more teriparatide exposure than humans showed an increase in osteosarcoma, a serious bone cancer, with use of teriparatide. This type of tumor is common in rats, but extremely rare in adult humans. For this reason, Health Canada limits its use to no more than 24 months over your lifetime. Talk with your doctor about your individual risk.

Things to consider

This is an option you may wish to discuss with your doctor if you are past menopause, have severe osteoporosis and fracture risk, and you have either tried other osteoporosis therapies without results or are unable to tolerate other medications. The cost of PTH is about $1000 per month so be sure to check your insurance coverage.

Table 17.7: Summary of Parathyroid Hormone

Medication and Brand Names	Pros	Cons
Parathyroid Hormone (Forteo)	Significant increase in BMD of the spine and moderate in the hip	Can use for a maximum of two years; expensive, $1000/month; Rare, but a concern, is bone cancer.

Bone builders not yet in North America

Strontium Ranelate

Strontium ranelate is a relatively new therapy for the treatment of postmenopausal osteoporosis. It is meant to reduce the risk of spinal and hip fractures in people with or without a previous history of fracture. It has not been released in the US or Canada (in 2009 the company that owns the patent to the drug's formula announced they would not be releasing it in Canada due to intellectual property rights issues).

How does strontium ranelate work on the bones?

Strontium ranelate is believed to have a dual action—increasing bone formation and reducing bone resorption, resulting in a rebalance of bone turnover in favor of bone formation.

Studies have shown an increase in bone strength and bone quality in both trabecular and cortical bone, the types of bone found in the vertebrae and hip respectively.

Strontium is a chemical element closely related to calcium, which can replace calcium in the bone. Strontium ranelate is composed of strontium and ranelic acid.

How well does strontium ranelate work on the bones?

Studies show strontium ranelate:

Reduces the risk of spinal fractures by 39% over 3 years

Reduces the risk of hip fracture by 15%.

Forms and dosing options

Strontium ranelate is marketed in Australia as Protos and under various names in other countries.

It is a once-daily dose, taken as a powder mixed with water. It is to be taken at bedtime, at least two hours after food, calcium-containing products, or antacids.

Possible side effects

• Blood clots

• Drug hypersensitivity syndrome which causes fever and/or rash and can affect other organs

• Nausea and diarrhea.

Things to consider

One drawback is that once treatment is stopped, the strontium is released fairly rapidly from the bone, unlike BPs.

Another concern is that the increase in BMD might be artificial because the strontium molecule is heavier than the calcium molecule. About half of the BMD increase may be attributed to the weight of the strontium itself.

Strontium ranelate is a new drug and therefore all of the risks and benefits of the long-term effects of the drug are unknown. Strontium does become incorporated into bone, and how that affects bone quality in the long-term is not clear.

Tibolone

Tibolone is a synthetic steroid hormone that mimics the effects of hormones produced by the ovaries. Tibolone is approved in Europe and many other countries, for the prevention of osteoporosis, but not in the US or Canada. One trial in 2006 concluded that Tibolone reduced the risk of fracture but the trial was halted due to increased incidence of stroke in older postmenopausal women with osteoporosis. The UK Million Women Study has found an increase in breast cancer with the use of any hormone-related therapy.

The drug is currently under review by the FDA in the US and will be sold under the trade name Xyvion if it is approved for use.

Parathyroid Hormone (PTH) 1-84

This is a synthetic version of parathyroid, marketed as Preos. It is administered as a daily injection. Research shows that it increases BMD and reduces the chances of spinal, but not hip, fractures.

Although studies show that it appears to be a safe and effective treatment option for osteoporosis, further trials are needed to determine its specific place in therapy compared with other treatment options.

Preos has been approved in Europe under the brand name Preotact and is being marketed by Nycomed as a treatment for osteoporosis in postmenopausal women at high risk of fractures. The name Preos and the new drug application is pending approval by the FDA in the United States. It is not clear what its future is in Canada.

Lasofoxifene (brand name Fablyn)

Lasofoxifene seemed to be a promising SERM under development by Pfizer for the prevention and treatment of osteoporosis. In 2005 the FDA did not approve it because of concerns that the drug might cause cancer in the lining of the uterus. The data were re-examined and Pfizer resubmitted it to the FDA in 2008 but again failed to win approval as clinical trials indicated that treatment with Fablyn led to an increase in deaths from stroke and cancer. The FDA advisory board determined that the drug's risks outweighed its benefits.

Some researchers claim Fablyn is the rare treatment that lowers the risk of both spinal and non-spinal fractures. Other researchers say it is merely a little more effective than Evista and that new agents should show clear benefits over existing agents.

In May 2010 Pfizer announced the withdrawal of its new drug application for Fablyn for the treatment of osteoporosis and selected consequences of menopause. However, Pfizer submitted applications to the European Medicines Agency (EMEA) for Fablyn for the treatment of osteoporosis in December 2007 and January 2008, respectively, and in February 2009, Pfizer received approval from the European Commission for Fablyn tablets.

It is not clear what the future of Fablyn is in North America.

Bazedoxifene (brand name Conbriza and Viviant)

Studies show that bazedoxifene, another SERM, significantly improved BMD at the spine and hip and reduced the risk of spinal fractures by about 40% in postmenopausal women with osteoporosis. It has no significant reduction on the of risk of hip fracture. Possible side effects include the risk of leg cramps and blood clots. The FDA declined to approve Viviant in 2008, saying it needed further analyses concerning the incidence of stroke and serious blood clots associated with the drug.

A Bone Builder for the Future

Odanacatib

Odanacatib inhibits an enzyme (cathepsin K) which is known to play a central role in the function of the cells that break down bone (osteoclasts).

Its mechanism of action differs from that of other antiresorptive agents. It does not reduce the number of osteoclasts and does not alter their function, thereby possibly offering theoretical advantages over bisphosphonates.

As of 2010, two studies have evaluated the efficacy and safety of odanacatib, a phase I study to determine the dose and a phase II study of safety and efficacy. Results of a phase II trial showed that a weekly dosage over 36 months resulted in increases in bone mineral density similar to those produced by other powerful antiresorptive drugs (zoledronate and denosumab). There are no data on fractures yet, a key element in demonstrating efficacy of a drug against osteoporosis. A study is ongoing with results expected in 2012.

Odanacatib could prove to be promising for osteoporosis patients looking for an alternative to bisphosphonates because of the possibility of undesirable effects over long-term use.

Generics

When a medication's patent expires and other companies are allowed to copy the formula, a generic brand may become available. Because the generic manufacturer does not have to recoup the cost of development and advertising, generic brands cost less than name brand medications.

Be aware that a generic medication may have a small but significant difference from the original brand that can create problems for some patients. Always ask your doctor or pharmacist about the safety of switching between brands of the same medication.

Nutritional Supplements

Many women want bone-building options without side effects so they turn to supplements in lieu of prescription medications. I am neither for or against these options. But there is little scientific evidence to support their claims and I find it challenging enough to choose between treatment options that have gone through extensive testing on thousands of women, let alone ingesting something that has not been sufficiently tested.

You can find supplements advertised on the internet that claim to prevent or even reverse osteoporosis. I urge you to be cautious in believing these claims. Many supplements offered on the internet and in health food stores have no evidence-based research to support their claims. Little is known about the risks and benefits of many of these supplements, so it is important to remember that a "natural" supplement may still have toxic side effects (mercury and poisonous mushrooms are both natural, after all).

Because nutritional supplements need not meet the rigorous standards that medications must, reputable scientific studies examining commercial non-prescription products are rare.

Drugs approved by Health Canada have:

- Been adequately studied and researched
- Proof of safety and efficacy
- Standard manufacturing and quality control
- Regulation of advertising claims.

But many natural health supplements have no:

- Adequate studies and research
- Proof of safety and efficacy
- Standard manufacturing and quality control
- Regulation of advertising claims.

Before taking any supplements:

- Talk to your doctor—among other concerns (cost, toxicity, etc.) it is important to know whether your supplement will act to increase or decrease the potency of any medical treatments you are taking

Check the label:

- Health Canada issues a product license after it has been assessed and found to be safe, effective, and of high quality under recommended conditions of use. Licensed natural health products in Canada have an eight-digit Natural Product Number (NPN) or Homeopathic Number (DIN-HM) on the label

Find a reputable pharmacist:

- There are pharmacists with expertise in natural products and homeopathic remedies.

Let's take a look at a few "bone-building" products I found offered on the internet.

Strontium

Supplements containing different forms and dosages of the mineral strontium are available in health food stores in Canada and the US. While small-scale independent trials with natural forms of strontium indicate a positive effect on bone health, only Servier's medicalized strontium ranelate, has gone through large-scale, double-blind random tests.

Natural health advocates believe that natural forms of the mineral can yield results similar to those obtained using strontium ranelate. However, experts say you cannot extrapolate data on strontium ranelate and apply it to nutritional supplements as the substances are different. Many osteoporosis organizations and doctors feel the jury is still out on strontium. They want to see studies showing the impact on bone from these strontium supplements.

OsteoDenx

OsteoDenx, available in US and Canada, from Nikken, claims to be a revolutionary formula that, according to the OsteoDenx website "supports natural bone tissue growth. It literally helps rebuild bone density." It then advises that these statements have not been evaluated by the Food and Drug Administration. The use of OsteoDenx is not supported by Osteoporosis Canada due to the lack of evidence-based research to support its claims. It is also quite expensive.

Good Vibrations Therapy–Step Up to the Plate to Build better Bones

Most miracle cures come into fashion and then disappear. Just visit the health section of a second hand book store if you want a reminder of the health trends of the last 30 to 40 years. Sometimes they are started by a true believer; sometimes they are started by a con artist exploiting the suffering of people who need a cure. So you can understand why I initially dismissed vibration therapy as another miracle cure that would not hold up to a bit of investigation.

Instead, I discovered that Canadian and American researchers are embarking on major clinical trials to see whether people with low bone density can vibrate their way to a healthier skeleton. There are people with osteoporosis who cannot tolerate any of the currently available medications. There are people whose fear of medication outweighs their fear of fracture. And there are those of us who would dearly love to find a non-drug therapy to improve our bone health. Depending on the research outcomes, vibration therapy may one day prove to be a promising option.

What is vibration therapy?

It is proven that placing stress on bone through exercise helps keep bones strong—and that lack of exercise causes bone loss. For example, astronauts who spend long periods without the earth's gravitational pressure lose two percent of their bone mass every month! Whole Body Vibration (WBV) was developed by the Russians in the 1970's to combat the problems of bone and muscle wasting in their cosmonauts as a result of spending time in zero gravity. The rapidly vibrating platform creates a form of hyper gravity that challenges the body to work harder. The result is a more effective and efficient physical training program.

There are two distinct types of machines on the market:

1. Whole Body Vibration Therapy (WBV) e.g., Galileo and PowerPlate.
2. Dynamic Motion Therapy (DMT).

At this point, the results are not in on whether vibration therapy helps bone health or is a dead end. There are concerns that the vibrations may cause fractures for people with very weak bones. Do not start this therapy without first discussing it with your doctor and evaluating risks and possible benefits.

How Whole Body Vibration Therapy (WBV) Works

Galileo is marketed as side-alternating vibration therapy. Once you step on the platform you will feel a natural unique side-alternating seesaw motion, which is very similar to the movement of walking, but with a lot less impact on your joints.

During conventional exercise our muscle movements are voluntary. But when using vibration therapy our muscles are stimulated to work by the involuntary stretch reflex (ISR), controlled by the spinal cord. The vibrating work stations resemble giant home scales with upraised handles.

The Galileo was developed first and is a tilting platform, to simulate the up-down and side-to-side action of the body during normal walking. This technology is patented (all other machines move vertically). A person stands on the tilting plate and a vibration comes through the plate. These vibrations are too fast for a person to voluntarily react to; however they stimulate the muscle, bone, and tendons which receive the vibration. Simply standing on the rapidly oscillating platform exercises the body's muscles and systems.

Things to consider

There have only been a few small studies examining the impact of WBV on bone in people with osteoporosis. There are issues about the safety of this vibration therapy in elderly people with a fragile skeleton and especially those who have broken bones easily. Further research is being conducted.

How Dynamic Motion Therapy (DMT) works

The DMT platform transmits high frequency, low intensity mechanical forces through a person's feet and up through the spine.

Small vibrations mimic what muscles cells do during common activities such as standing, maintaining balance, and walking. They twitch in a sequence of tiny contractions that exert small stresses on the bone said to result in new bone formation. The up-and-down movement of the Juvent Platform no bigger than the width of a few human hairs. So the motion is said to be gentle.

Juvent claims that maximum benefit is reached when the platform is used at least five days a week for 10 to 20 minutes each day. Claims state that you can simply stand on the platform and read or watch television.

Things to consider

As with WBV, there have only been a few small studies examining the impact of DMT on bone in people with osteoporosis.

Scientists are studying the benefits of a vibration therapy by putting volunteers through workouts on vibrating platforms. The goal is to to offer an alternative or complementary therapy to help build bone with a workout program that is safe and practical.

"There is preliminary data suggesting that these machines (Juvent 1000 DMT platform) may have potential benefits for bones," says Dr. Angela Cheung, director of the osteoporosis program for the University Health Network and Mount Sinai Hospital in Toronto. She is hoping that the benefit to the bone will be similar to calcium and vitamin D supplementation.

The Juvent 1000 (approximate cost $3,000) has already been licensed as a medical device by health Canada.

Warning

Do not confuse the Galileo and Juvent platforms (devices created specifically for osteoporosis treatment) with other vibration machines designed to increase muscle-tone, balance, and weight loss. These machines, such as the Power Plate, are used for athletic conditioning and have a much stronger vibration—one that can damage bone and even cause a fracture.

CHAPTER 18

~

PREVENTING FALL-RELATED FRACTURES

When bones are weak a simple fall can lead to a fracture. Preventing falls is important at any age, but it is especially important for those who have osteoporosis because our bones are more fragile and easily broken.

Each year, a third of people who are 65 years of age or older will fall. Some will be permanently disabled by the broken bones that can follow. The risk of falling increases with age and is greater for women than for men.

Falls contribute to fractures of the wrist, spine, pelvis, or hip. The most common osteoporotic fracture is the spinal fracture but the most debilitating is a hip fracture. 90% of broken hips come from falls. Factors that increase your risk of falling are:

- You are over the age of 65

- You take medication to help you sleep or calm your nerves

- You take multiple medications per day

- You have problems with balance or difficulty walking

- You have difficulty getting in or out of the bathtub unassisted

- You have problems with strength or sensation in your legs or feet

- You have chronic pain

- You have had a slip, trip, or fall in the last 12 months.

There are three factors that play a role in breaking a bone. If one of these factors is changed, the chances of breaking a bone are greatly reduced. The three factors are:

1. Fall: the fall itself.
2. Force: the force and direction of the fall.
3. Fragility: the fragility of the bones that take the impact.

Fall: the Fall Itself

The best way to prevent an injury from a fall is NOT to fall. Most falls take place in the home—and what might be a painful bruise without osteoporosis can become a crippling injury if our bones are weak.

Here is a simple checklist to adopt to reduce the chance of a fall in your home:

1. Talk to your doctor and pharmacist about your medications and supplements and any possible interactions or side effects— dizziness, drowsiness, muscle spasms, etc., can all contribute to a fall.

2. Install grab bars for the bath tub and shower. Be sure to have a full length rubber mat in the tub or non-skid tape and a non-skid bath mat bedside the tub. Add non-skid tape to the shower floor.

3. Keep floors and stairs free of clutter. Remove small throw rugs. Make sure carpets are anchored and smooth (no bubbles) to prevent tripping.

4. Landscape walkways to ensure they are level.

5. Ensure you have hand rails for all stairways in and outside of the home, preferably on both sides of the stairway.

6. Install support poles or rails to make it easier to get in and out of bed.

7. Add non-slip stair tread coverings.

8. Add firm foam to seat cushions to make it easier to get in and out of chairs and sofas (prevents "sinking" into furniture).

9. Install proper lighting in the home especially at the top and bottom of the stairways and be sure to have a night-light near the washroom.

10. Wear comfortable non-slip footwear in the home and avoid wearing socks or stockings that are slippery, especially on wood floors.

11. Install non-slip flooring in the kitchen and bathrooms.

12. Remove or hide all loose wires and cords i.e., around the computer or tape wires to the wall.

13. Add a non-skid mat in the kitchen and clean up spills right away!

14. Slow down! Try not to be in a rush especially on the stairs.

15. Keep the items you use often within easy reach (on shelves at waist level).

16. Don't take chances. Know your limitations. Think twice if what you are about to do is risky (i.e., climbing up to the top of a stepladder to get a heavy box from a cupboard). Ask for help if you need it!

Force & Direction

Sometimes, there's no way to avoid a fall. With that in mind, you can at least prepare properly to fall. You have less than two seconds from the moment you slip until you hit the ground. That's precious little time to react. Knowing how to fall will help you reduce the risk of fracture. Let's take a look at how to cushion a fall to lessen the impact on your bones. Review these suggestions with your physiotherapist to help you prevent injuries.

How hard you fall plays a major role in determining whether or not a fracture will occur. The greater the distance an individual has to fall, the greater the force of the impact.

Essentially, if you land on just one body point (say the hand or hip), then all impact forces converge on that point—and then go right into your body. The fewer parts of the body that hit the ground, the larger hit each one of those parts must take. You want to try to spread the impact across your body or, on your whole forearm as opposed to just your wrist.

The angle at which the individual falls is also important because it can channel even more force into one of your bone danger zones. Falling sideways or straight down is more risky than falling backwards.

Falling Sideways

- If falling to the left or right you want your forearm (not your wrist, shoulder, or hip) to be the first to contact the floor
- Try to break the fall with your whole forearm as opposed to just your hand
- If falling to the left, keep the left arm bent and try to break the fall with your left forearm
- If falling to the right, keep the right arm bent and try to break the fall with your right forearm
- Also, lift your head toward your shoulder opposite the fall.

Falling Backwards

- Make sure you bend your knees
- Tuck your chin in to your chest to break your fall
- Extend your arms away from your body and slap the ground with your palms and forearms at about a 45 degree angle.

Falling Forward

- Bend your left knee
- Throw your right leg back
- Orient your hands in the shape of a triangle with palms down and turn your head to the side so your face does not hit the ground
- Hands should be flush to the ground.

Fragility of the Bones Taking the Impact

The more fragile our bones, the more likely they are to be damaged by the force of a fall. Previous chapters have covered how you can help your bone health with nutrition, medication (if necessary), and exercise. In this case, exercises that build and strengthen muscles in both the back and legs will make you more sure-footed and less likely to have a damaging fall.

When thinking about fracture prevention don't discount the risk of falls and their consequences. This is one area where you can play a key role in being fracture free.

CHAPTER 19

YOUR BONE-BUILDING TEAM

Managing osteoporosis requires the coordinated care of your health care team. Doctors, nurses, and other members of your osteoporosis team help provide a piece to the overall puzzle to enable you to live well with osteoporosis. I was blessed with a team of knowledgeable and compassionate men and women who, to this day, assist and encourage me in managing osteoporosis instead of letting osteoporosis manage me!

Build a Bone-building Team

Here is a list of the types of professionals that were an integral part of my bone-building team. Women with osteoporosis might also include psychologists / psychiatrists (or other types of mental health therapists), acupuncturists, holistic practitioners, etc., on their teams. There are many physical and emotional challenges to overcome when living with osteoporosis, especially after the tough changes that fractures create in daily life.

Table 19.1

Title	Role
General practitioner/ physician/family doctor	Doctor who provides primary care. Diagnosis and management of the disease. Should include: fracture risk assessment, ordering tests (i.e., bone density and blood work), and prescription for medications if required.
Physical therapy- physiotherapistor osteopathic manual practitioner	Physical therapist with experience in osteoporosis. Educate, improve posture, strength, flexibility, well being, and pain management.
Occupational Therapy	A health professional with experience in osteoporosis who helps people regain the ability to perform the activities of daily life.

Title	Role
Personal Trainer/ Wellness Coach	Exercise coach with experience in osteoporosis. Design a healthy exercise program tailored to meet your individual needs to gain strength and flexibility and prevent future fractures. Help set goals and encourage you to stay motivated to exercise.
Dietitian	Nutrition check up. Healthy diet advice about calcium, vitamin D and other important nutrients you can get in your diet to improve your overall health.
Dentist	Maintain and work to keep gums, teeth and jawbone healthy. Monitor dental health especially when on bisphosphonates.
Pharmacist	Pharmaceutical care of osteoporotic patients. Ensure safe and effective use of medications and help patients achieve healthier outcomes from medication therapy. Advice when taking prescription medication and help when choosing calcium and vitamin D supplements if required.
Massage therapist	With experience in osteoporosis. Relaxation, reduce muscle spasms and tension and pain management.
Image consultant, hair stylist, esthetician	Help regain your confidence and self-image after the effects of spinal fractures. Help choosing clothing and hairstyle to enhance your personal appearance. Help with pedicures if bending to reach your toes is difficult after spinal fractures. Pamper yourself!
Family and friends	Good listeners who provide support and motivation, along with practical help when you ask for it.
National osteoporosis organizations and local support groups	Continuous learning about advances and research in bone health, medication options, exercises, and a chance to share experiences and learn from others living with osteoporosis.

Physician

A physician looks at your total health care from the tips of your toes to the top of your head. To diagnose patients with diseases such as osteoporosis, they will often request tests that include a bone density test and blood work—in 2000, 80% of Canadian bone mineral density scans were ordered by family physicians rather than specialists. In Canada, family physicians provide diagnosis, treatment, and advocacy on behalf of patients. They have particular skills in treating people with multiple health issues.

Physicians can help provide you with a meaningful report on your bone density results, compare it to previous BMDs, and help you understand your fracture risk. They discuss when to start treatment, what medication options are available, which might be best for you, and how you and your bone health will be monitored.

Your physician provides credible information and advice to improve your bone health and coordinate communication and tests to and from specialists when necessary.

Physician's team

A physician may have a team of people supporting her to help her carry out her role more effectively including a receptionist, nurse, nurse practitioner, or resident.

- A *nurse practitioner* is a registered nurse with advanced education and training who can treat patients in collaboration with physicians
- A *resident* has completed an MD and practices medicine under the supervision of a fully licensed physician helping to provide patient care.

The specific duties of these team players vary depending on the types of duties that the supervising physician chooses to assign. These team players may: conduct patient interviews, take medical histories, and provide counseling on preventive health care.

How to get the most out of your doctor's visit

Do your homework before the visit to your doctor (see Chapter 4). Prioritize your concerns and be aware that you may not be able to address all of them in one visit—you won't have a lot of time, so be concise. I find doctors appreciate patients who come prepared.

1. Be organized and write down your top three questions.

2. Be respectful and kind to the nurses, assistants, medical students in training, and receptionists. They are often overworked and they help get you in the door to see the doctor, so treat them well!

Physiotherapist or Osteopathic Manual Practitioner

Physical therapists (physiotherapists or osteopathic manual practitioners) offer guidance on safe exercises and activities. Physical therapists can help patients with posture, body mechanics and safe movement. They can also perform balance assessment and training that is important for preventing falls. (See Chapter 10 for a more complete explanation of osteopathic manual practitioners and physiotherapists.)

A credible physiotherapist or osteopathic manual practitioner will help you:

- Maintain bone strength
- Prevent fractures
- Improve muscle strength, balance, and cardiovascular fitness
- Improve posture
- Improve psychological well-being
- Aim to reduce falls
- Help relieve pain, fear and anxiety
- Give lifestyle advice on lifting and handling, posture, and safe exercise/activity.

Occupational Therapist

Occupational therapists address activities of daily living and upper body function. The focus is on preserving your independence. Occupational therapy provides retraining in bathing, grooming, dressing, toileting, meal preparation, and housekeeping.

Occupational therapy practitioners will help you create a fall prevention program. To understand a client's capabilities, the practitioner might ask the client to perform some typical activities, such as climbing stairs or getting in and out of the bathtub and then suggest new ways to do things and/or recommend adaptive equipment.

Physicians and other medical professionals can refer you to occupational therapy practitioners in your area. Other sources for locating an occupational therapist include colleagues, family members, and friends who have received occupational therapy services, as well as your local telephone directory.

Professional Life & Wellness Coach

In pain from my fractures and fearing the future, I didn't have much motivation to start and sustain an exercise program. This is where my wellness coach came in. Find one who has knowledge of the challenges of osteoporosis and can help you set goals and create programs tailored for your individual personality.

We aimed to create small changes that delivered results—I found my coach so helpful that I continue to use her services even now. With her encouragement and support we created a program that has helped me stay active and has increased my ability to enjoy activities with my husband, daughter, family, and friends. It also helped improve my self-confidence and feeling of being better able to manage my osteoporosis. We revise my program as I become stronger.

My wellness coach had the knowledge and expertise to assess my diet and recommend important changes to help maintain and even enhance my health. Some women choose to seek the advice of a dietitian.

Dietitian

Dietitians are health professionals whose knowledge and expertise in food and nutrition support people to make healthy food choices. This is even more important when dealing with something like osteoporosis. Good nutrition plays an important role in promoting wellness and vitality as well as reducing the risks of osteoporosis, heart disease, different types of cancer, diabetes, and other conditions. Dietary factors affect the passage of calcium in and out of the bones. Your dietitian can help you create shopping lists, menus, and even find recipes that include foods rich in calcium, vitamin D, and other important nutrients. In addition, your dietitian will help you create a diet low in foods that hurt bone density such as soft drinks (phosphorus), caffeine, alcohol, and salt.

Your doctor should be able to recommend a dietitian who is knowledgeable in bone health.

Dentist

The jawbone is connected to all those bones below our neck. Something as routine as an oral exam and x-ray can reveal a decrease in bone density and your dentist may refer you to your physician for medical assessment. Research shows bone health may be connected with the health of our jawbone, teeth, and even our gums.

Because weak bone can accelerate gum disease and, conversely, gum disease can break down weak bones, your dentist may be the first person to suspect you have osteoporosis.

Few people consider tooth loss when faced with the possibility of osteoporosis. Because your jaw is made of bone and holds your teeth in place, they can fall out if osteoporosis weakens your jaw bone. To help preserve your smile make it a point to visit your dentist regularly and talk to your dentist about osteoporosis and your bone health. Simple, regular cleanings by your dentist or dental hygienist could eliminate the periodontal disease that accelerates bone and tooth loss.

Remember that your oral health affects your overall health and vice versa. Special attention should be given to all patients on bisphosphonate therapy. In my view, they should receive maximum attention to prevent dental problems and maintain their oral health. Dentists should consider referring these patients to a specialist for even the simplest necessary extraction or other dental surgical procedures to manage the serious adverse effects that may arise from oral surgery.

Pharmacist

Your pharmacist can be integral to the management of your osteoporosis. He or she is usually easily accessible and can be a reliable source of information about osteoporosis medications, and the right vitamin and mineral supplements for your condition. She or he can help you monitor your condition, maximize the benefits of your medications, limit side effects, and identify drug interactions.

When I have questions about my medications I consult with a pharmacist to review my prescriptions. It is an opportunity to learn more about different aspects of my medications. This can include more information about when to take medications to increase their effectiveness, or reduce side effects, and development of strategies to manage your medication schedule and ensure medications are not missed.

A good pharmacist will encourage you to get involved with your health care. Studies have found that patients who work with their pharmacists to manage their medications and health have:

- Lower health care costs
- Fewer trips to emergency departments
- Fewer hospitalizations
- Fewer problems caused by medications
- A better understanding of how to take their medications
- Better management of health conditions like osteoporosis.

If you have questions and concerns about your medication, possible side effects and how long to take the treatment, I suggest you raise these with your pharmacist. Local pharmacists can offer additional support by providing contact information for a local support group.

Massage Therapist

When a vertebra breaks, some people have no pain, while others have intense pain and muscle spasms that last long after the fracture has healed. A qualified massage therapist with experience in osteoporosis can help relieve pain, relax stiff muscles, and smooth out muscle knots by increasing the blood supply to the affected area and warming it. If you have osteoporosis, don't allow a therapist to deep massage near your spine. The pressure can cause fractures. Light, circular massage with fingers or the palm of the hand is best in this case.

Image Consultant

Besides the obvious challenges I faced because of my spinal fractures, I experienced consistent frustration in my daily efforts to look good and feel better about myself. I was discouraged by all the changes to my physique, including the loss of height after the spinal fractures. After advice from an image consultant, I know what hairstyles, clothes, and colours best help my new proportions and help me feel happy when I catch a glimpse of myself in the mirror. When we look good, we feel good!

Esthetician

I was no longer able to care for my feet because I couldn't bend that far without risking pain, or even fracture. I treat myself to a monthly pedicure—it takes care of some potentially painful foot problems like cracked heels and ingrown nails before they develop. Perhaps more importantly, it's a time when I enjoy my body with a pampering experience that leaves me feeling good. My esthetician knows my challenges and is always careful to make sure that I have the back support I need.

Hairstylist

We all know the expression "bad hair day." Well, when you are down and discouraged a hair cut and colour can often cheer you up! And the "kind ear" provided by hairstylists can be an important source of informal social support.

My stylist has gone above and beyond, looking after my hair in the hospital and at home when I was too incapacitated to travel to her salon.

If some of these services are not within your budget choose the ones that are most important. Also, when friends and family ask for your gift preferences, mention how much you would like a gift certificate that you could use towards these services.

Family & Friends

The support and love from my husband and daughter is indescribable. They are patient, loving, and understanding. I am also fortunate to have many incredible family members and dear friends who have provided support and encouragement since my spinal fractures. Having a friend or family member who is living with a chronic disease and/or with pain is challenging. I find the friends and family members most helpful who:

- Are willing to learn a bit about osteoporosis

- Don't assume they know how I feel. My days can be unpredictable; some days I feel great and others are painful. If you have never lived a day with a spinal fracture yourself, you don't know how the person is feeling. Just because I am not crying or visibly in pain, it does not mean I am not suffering silently

- Are a good listener. Osteoporosis causes frustration. There is a physical, emotional, social, and financial impact associated with my spinal fractures. I try to be positive but some days are over-whelming and I just need to vent!

- Are adaptable—sometimes I need to sit in the firmest chair in the room or take the guest room that has the firmest bed, etc. So I just ask that people understand why I have these needs. I am not being needlessly picky!

- Offer unconditional love and friendship. My family and friends know I have new limitations and different needs, but I still treasure my family relationships and friendships.

Osteoporosis Canada (OC) & the National Osteoporosis Foundation (NOF) (US)

OC and the NOF are valuable sources of information and support. Be sure to look at their sites weekly to get up-to-date information on educational seminars, treatment options, and events in your city. Get involved as a volunteer or speaker or advocate or join the Canadian Osteoporosis Patient Network (COPN) or a Strong Bones Peer Support Group or initiate one in your community.

Strong Bones Peer Support Group

If fractures caused by osteoporosis affect you as an individual, they will also affect your family.

Professionals who help people deal with loss have long used the five stages of acceptance as a kind of roadmap to help people proceed with living their lives as normally as possible, or at least, to help them recognize where they are in the grieving process. This "roadmap" was originally intended for dealing with grief. In the case of a chronic disease such as osteoporosis, this grieving can be for the loss of our own expectation of good health. For the rest of your family, it is the loss of you as a normal, healthy individual within the family.

Being aware of the stages can be a useful tool to describe the process in a way that is easily understood. You can have ups and down emotionally as you continue through life with chronic disease, and you might sometimes go backwards or forwards towards acceptance. This is normal. The five stages are simply convenient shorthand for describing a process that we and our families go through.

The five stages are denial, anger, bargaining, depression, and acceptance. We all eventually learn to live with whatever diseases we have. Acceptance is knowing that, while we don't choose osteoporosis and we would prefer not to have it, with proper treatment and perhaps with lifestyle changes, we can live a good life and prevent future fractures even though we may have some limitations we didn't have before. Some people reach acceptance quickly; others take some time to get there. Sometimes it can be useful to be able to talk to someone other than family and friends (who may not truly understand what we are going through). This could be a member of your health care team, a member of your church, or a support group.

There is no better place to gain understanding than from a group of people who live with osteoporosis. The interaction with a larger group offers you a broader scope of understanding, especially since not all people with osteoporosis have identical effects after fractures, undergo the same treatments, or cope the same way. We can learn from each other and from shared experiences.

For People with Osteoporosis: How to Find a Doctor

For many people, finding a doctor who is knowledgeable about osteoporosis can be challenging. There is no physician specialty dedicated solely to osteoporosis. A variety of medical specialists treat people with osteoporosis, including family doctors, endocrinologists, rheumatologists, gynecologists, orthopedic surgeons, and geriatricians.

There are a number of ways to find a doctor who treats osteoporosis patients. If you have a primary care or family doctor, discuss your concerns with him or her. Your doctor may treat the disease or be able to refer you to an osteoporosis specialist.

Over time, some healthcare providers in different medical specialties have gained the knowledge and expertise to diagnose and treat people with osteoporosis. These specialties include endocrinology, rheumatology, geriatrics, gynecology, and orthopedics. However, not all healthcare providers within a given specialty have expertise in osteoporosis.

There are a number of ways to find a healthcare provider who treats patients with osteoporosis. If you have a primary care physician or family doctor, discuss your concerns with him or her first. You may find that your own healthcare provider is quite knowledgeable about osteoporosis. If not, your doctor may be able to refer you to someone who specializes in osteoporosis.

If you do not have a personal doctor or if your doctor cannot help, contact OC or the NOF. They can direct you to a local support group and they may be able to suggest a doctor in your community. Or try the nearest university hospital and ask for the department that cares for patients with osteoporosis. Some hospitals have a separate osteoporosis program or clinic that treats patients with osteoporosis. Your own primary care doctor—whether a physician or gynecologist—is often the best person to treat you because she or he knows your medical history, your lifestyle, and your special needs.

Medical Specialists Who Treat Osteoporosis

After an initial assessment, it may be necessary to see an endocrinologist, a rheumatologist, or another specialist to rule out the possibility of an underlying disease that may contribute to osteoporosis.

Do I need to see a specialist?

Most osteoporosis is cared for by physicians. But if any of the following are true, your physician may refer you to an endocrinologist or rheumatologist:

1. You have osteoporosis at a young age—premenopausal.
2. Your osteoporosis is not well managed despite your physician's efforts. (i.e., your bone density continues to decline).
3. Your physician is not well versed in the most recent information about osteoporosis management and medications.
4. Despite attempts to manage your osteoporosis, you have another fracture.
5. You have a suspected or known condition that may underlie the osteoporosis (i.e., hyperthyroidism).

Waiting times for consultations with specialists in Canada can be several months or more. Due to the shortage of specialists, physicians consider seriously before making a referral. In my case, because of my relative youth and the severity of my bone loss, I was referred to a specialist very early in my treatment.

Endocrinologists

Endocrinologists treat the endocrine system, which includes the glands and hormones that help control the body's metabolic activity.

In addition to osteoporosis, conditions often treated by endocrinologists include diabetes, thyroid disorders and pituitary diseases.

It is a physician's prerogative to refer the patient for consultation to qualified experts. Osteoporosis is a complex endocrinologic disorder of bone and mineral metabolism. An endocrinologist is a reliable resource for primary physicians who seek consultation for their patients with osteoporosis and other metabolic bone diseases.

Rheumatologists

Rheumatologists specialize in the diagnosis, management, and treatment of musculoskeletal (joints, muscles, bones, and tendons) diseases. Osteoporosis is an important member of this family of diseases. Expertise in osteoporosis is an important professional focus of many rheumatologists.

Rheumatologists have a practice structure that emphasizes detailed analysis of complex medical problems. They have the skills to interpret bone density measurement and other factors key to diagnosing and following patients with osteoporosis.

Geriatricians

These family doctors or internists have received additional training on the aging process and the conditions and diseases that often occur among the elderly, including incontinence, falls, and dementia. Geriatricians often care for patients in nursing homes, in patients' homes, or in office or hospital settings.

Gynecologists

These physicians diagnose and treat conditions of the female reproductive system and associated disorders. They often serve as primary care doctors for women and follow their patients' reproductive health over time.

Orthopedic Surgeons

These doctors are trained in the care of patients with musculo-skeletal conditions, such as congenital skeletal malformations, bone fractures and infections, and metabolic problems. They are surgeons who operate to correct, fix or replace joints and limbs.

Who is the most Most Important Member of Your Bone-building Team?

You! To quote Senator Wilbert Keon, heart surgeon, founder of the University of Ottawa Heart Institute and member of the senate sub-committee on population health: "50% of the disease that's being treated in the health-care delivery system is preventable. We have people living in such unhealthy circumstances that they can't possibly be healthy, no matter how good the health-care delivery system is. In essence, the health care delivery system is responsible for about 25% of outcomes, and 75% of health outcomes are the result of your genetic predisposition plus all the social determinants of health."

Your health care team can only do so much. You must be the pivotal member of the team... the conductor or quarterback. Doctors have limited time and competing demands during appointments. You need to be assertive (not aggressive) in making your needs known and your concerns heard. You are in the best position to know your own needs.

Staying on top of current therapies for preventing and treating osteoporosis presents a challenge for busy practitioners. So you need to be aware of new treatments and prompt your physician to explore them with you.

You may need to be the information gatekeeper to help improve communication between your physician and other health care team members with respect to your follow-up, medication, and tests to ensure top osteoporosis management. Keep a file and log all your appointments, medications and outcomes. It is in your interest to do so.

In order to live well with osteoporosis we must play a key role in our bone health. We cannot sit on the sidelines and rely on others to do it for us. We must not only be an active participant but a key player.

CHAPTER 20

~

PARTING WORDS

Osteoporosis broke some of my bones but it did not break my spirit.

There came a point when I wanted to turn my life around and get well. I scoured bookstores and libraries to find information on how to manage this disease. I quickly became frustrated, as I found very few books and those that I did find had a mere paragraph or two on spinal fractures. Most books focused on prevention of bone loss and glossed over details of fractures and pain. I sought out health professionals with knowledge about osteoporosis and questioned them at length. I contacted what is now called Osteoporosis Canada. I accumulated an entire room full of material. My research, along with my own journey, is this book.

Over the years that I compiled my research the media have increased coverage of chronic diseases, such as osteoporosis, due to our aging population in North America. Also, the internet has a plethora of articles on weak bones. A quick search on Google led to 1,500,000 results! For someone suffering from osteoporosis, it can be overwhelming to sort out what is fact, what is fiction, or just plain misleading advertising. As I struggled to get the right information to make important decisions about my bone health, I did the research for you—so you can review it and make use of it with your health care team.

My road to recovery after spinal fractures and learning to live with osteoporosis was anything but a direct route. The journey has been both a physical and emotional one. And I questioned whether I was ever going to emerge from the despair and pain after my spinal fractures. But I did. I am hoping that this book has helped you avoid the agony and uncertainty that I endured by not knowing much about the disease—and, more importantly, the consequences of a fracture. I hope that after reading this book you know that you can and will improve. But it will take patience and persistence.

A passive reading of this book will prove disappointing. You must be an active participant, which means you are in for a lot of work. Real changes in your bone health can only be achieved through:

- Good nutrition (especially calcium and vitamin D)
- The right exercises and activities to strengthen your muscles and bones
- Medication (if necessary)
- Doing your homework prior to your medical appointments
- Being an active participant with your health care team.

It is also helpful to remember the mind-body connection. Consider options such as meditation and relaxation techniques and participating in a support group to talk to others who have been through what you are going through and have overcome hurdles living with osteoporosis.

Whew! Sounds daunting. The key is baby steps and to give yourself permission to vary from any expected norms. Accept your own rate of progression to build better bones, especially after a spinal fracture. We are all unique. Be sure to celebrate your successes and thank all of those people who have helped you along the way.

I have learned so much from my experiences and journey living with osteoporosis and spinal fractures. Although I am not happy to have this disease, I am so grateful for the support and encouragement I have received from so many people especially my husband and daughter, my other family members, friends, and Osteoporosis Canada.

The future for better bone health is promising. The research to determine the best strategies for osteoporosis prevention and care is growing. The number of people advocating for better bone health through organizations around the world such as Osteoporosis Canada and the National Osteoporosis Foundation is encouraging. And as proceeds from the sale of this book go to Osteoporosis Canada, your purchase will help further OC's efforts. New medications to treat osteoporosis are being developed and tested, giving patients more options to choose from to better their bone health and live an active life.

Being diagnosed with osteoporosis does not mean you have to suffer with poor bone health the rest of your life. You will, however, have to make the effort to help yourself. Osteoporosis cannot be cured but it can be managed and you can live well with the disease.

My life has changed and I am always conscious of the fact that I could have another broken bone, but I am much more confident and I get joy and pleasure out of life.

I wrote this book partly to provide women with more insight into this potentially debilitating disease and encourage you to do some "bone health" homework. But my real desire is to provide hope, inspiration and tools to help you manage osteoporosis and not let it manage you.

My parting thoughts are simple:

Be good to your bones and your bones will be good to you!

REFERENCES & RESOURCES

Below is a list of references and resources I used as I researched and wrote *Unbreakable*. Most are available online so I have added the websites for easy access to additional information.

Introduction and Chapter 1

Facts and statistics. International Osteoporosis Foundation, 2009.
http://www.iofbonehealth.org

Fast facts. National Osteoporosis Foundation, 2010.
http://www.nof.org/node/40

How many people are affected by osteoporosis? Timeless Women, 2009.
http://www.fortimelesswomen.com

Osteoporosis at-a-glance. Osteoporosis Canada, 2010.
http://www.osteoporosis.ca/index.php/ci_id/5526/la_id/1.htm

Chapter 2

2010 Clinical Practice Guidelines, for the Diagnosis and Management of Osteoporosis in Canada, CMAJ, Oct. 12, 2010.
http://www.cmaj.ca/home/review.dtl or http://www.osteoporosis.ca

Building strong bones for a lifetime. University of Arizona, 2006.
http://ag.arizona.edu/maricopa/fcs/bb/index.htm

Canadian Multicentre Osteoporosis Study. http://www.camos.org

Chapuy M et al. "Vitamin D3 and calcium to prevent hip fractures in elderly women." *N Eng J Med* 1992:327:1637-42.
http://www.nejm.org/doi/pdf/10.1056/nejm199212033272305

Exercising with osteoporosis: Stay active the safe way. Mayo Clinic.
http://www.mayoclinic.com/health/osteoporosis/HQ00643

Facts and statistics about osteoporosis and its impact. International Osteoporosis Foundation, 2010. http://www.iofbonehealth.org.

Ho, SC et al. "Determinants of peak bone mass in Chinese and Caucasian populations." *HKMJ* 1995;1:38-42.
http://www.hkmj.org/article_pdfs/hkm9503p38.pdf

National Osteoporosis Foundation. http://www.nof.org

Osteoporosis Australia. http://www.osteoporosis.org

Physical activity, 2010. Osteoporosis Canada.
http://www.osteoporosis.ca

Sherrer Y et al. *Osteoporosis, A Woman Doctor's Guide, Prevent and Reverse Bone Loss at Any Age*, New York, N.Y. Kensington Publishing, 2001.

Zmuda JM. "Identification of osteoporosis risk genes: The tip of the iceberg." *Ann Intern Med*, 2009;151:581-582.
http://www.annals.org/content/151/8/581.full.pdf+html

Chapter 3 and Chapter 4
2010 Clinical Practice Guidelines, for the Diagnosis and Management of Osteoporosis in Canada, CMAJ, Oct. 12, 2010.
http://www.cmaj.ca/home/review.dtl or http://www.osteoporosis.ca

Bernstein C et al. "The incidence of fracture among patients with inflammatory bowel disease: a population-based cohort study." *Annals Int Med*, Nov. 21, 2000 133:795-799.
http://www.annals.org/cgi/content/abstract/133/10/795

Binkley N. "Summary - The role of vitamin D in musculoskeletal health." *J Musculoskelet Neuronal Interact* 2006; 6(4):347-348.
http://www.ismni.org/jmni/pdf/26/15BINKLEY_summary.pdf

Canadian Diabetes Association, 2009. http://www.diabetes.ca:80/about-diabetes/what

Clark MK et al. "Bone mineral density and fractures among alcohol-dependent women in treatment and in recovery." *Osteoporosis Int.*, 2003;14:396-403.

Chron's and Osteoporosis, 2009. http://colitis.emedtv.com/crohn's-disease/crohn's-and-osteoporosis.html

Clinician's Guide to Prevention and Treatment of Osteoporosis, 2010. National Osteoporosis Foundation.
http://www.nof.org/professionals/clinical-guidelines

Connection between depression and osteoporosis shown by Hebrew University researchers, 2009.
http://www.hunews.huji.ac.il/articles.asp?artID=692&cat=6

Cummings SR et al. "Epidemiology of osteoporosis and osteoporotic fractures." *Epidemiol Rev* 1985;7:178-208.

Cummings SR et al. "Bone density at various sites for prediction of hip fracture." The Study of Osteoporotic Fractures Research group. *Lancet* 1993; 341:72-5.

Delmas et al. "The use of biochemical markers of bone turnover in osteoporosis." *Osteoporosis Int.*, 2000(Suppl 6): S2-17.

Dental Wellness Institute, 2009.
http://dentalwellness4u.com/dentaldisease/osteoporosis.html

Depression among the risk factors for osteoporosis. Harvard Women's Health Watch, 2010.
https://www.health.harvard.edu/press_releases/depression-osteoporosis

Diagnosis. T score. International Osteoporosis Foundation.
http://www.iofbonehealth.org/patients-public/about-osteoporosis/diagnosis.html

El-Hajj FG et al. Editors. "Practice guidelines on the use of bone mineral density measurements. Who to test? What measures to use? When to treat? A consensus report from the Middle East Densitometry Workshop." *Lebanese Medical Journal* 2002; 50 (3): 89.
http://staff.aub.edu.lb/~webcmop/manuscript/HF%202002.pdf

Endo Resolved, Treatment Options for Endometriosis, 2010.
http://www.endo-resolved.com/treatment.html

Eustice C et al. "The rheumatoid arthritis-osteoporosis link."
About.com, 2006.
http://arthritis.about.com/od/rheumatoidarthritis/a/osteoporosis.htm

Facts and statistics about osteoporosis and its impact. International Osteoporosis Foundation. http://www.iofbonehealth.org/facts-and-statistics.html

Felsenberg, D et al. "The Bone Quality Framework: Determinants of Bone Strength and Their Interrelationships, and Implications for Osteoporosis Management." *Clinical Therapeutics*, 2005;27:1:1-11.
http://www.sciencedirect.com/

Frax®, WHO fracture risk assessment tool.
http://www.sheffield.ac.uk/FRAX/

Hayes WC et al. "Impact near the hip dominates fracture risk in elderly nursing home residents who fall." *Calcif Tissue Int* 1993;52:192-198.

Hawker G. "Bone biology and the investigation of osteoporosis." *J Soc Obstet Gynaecol* Can 1996; 18 (July suppl): 1-6.

Holick, M. "The role of vitamin D in the management of osteoporosis." 2009. (Slides With Audio). http://cme.medscape.com/viewarticle/ 588246

Potential affects of Depo-Provera on bone mineral density in adults and adolescents-Pfizer Canda Inc., Health Canada. 2005. http://www.hc-sc.gc.ca/dhp-mps/medeff/advisoriesavis/prof/_2005/ depo-provera_2_hpc-cps-eng.php

Jabbour S. Systemic Effects of Oral Glucocorticoids, MedscapeCME, 2006. http://cme.medscape.com/viewarticle/549746

Kung, A. "The effect of thyroid hormone on bone metabolism and osteoporosis." *J Hong Kong Med Assoc* 1994;46:3:249.

Leibson et al. "Mortality, disability, and nursing home use for persons with and without hip fracture: a population-based study." *J of American Geriatrics Society* 2002;50:1644–50.

Magaziner J et al. "Recovery from hip fracture in eight areas of function." *Journal of Gerontology: Medical Sciences* 2000;55A(9):M498–507.

Multiple Sclerosis Society of Canada, 2009.
http://www.mssociety.ca/en/information/default.htm

National Institute of Arthritis and Musculoskeletal and Skin Diseases, 2009. http://www.niams.nih.gov/health_info/bone/Osteoporosis/ Conditions_Behaviors/diabetes.asp

NIH consensus development panel on osteoporosis, prevention, diagnosis and therapy. JAMA 2001;285:785. http://jama.ama-assn.org/cgi/content/abstract/285/6/785

Nelson, M et al. *Strong Women Strong Bones, everything you need to know to prevent, treat, and beat osteoporosis*, Penguin Group, New York, NY, 2000, p 72-76.

Oncology Resource Centre, 2009. http://patient.cancerconsultants.com/ Osteoporosis Update, A Practical Guide for Physicians, Winter 2003 vol. 7, no.1.

Osteoporosis Update, Secondary causes of osteoporosis, Fall 2007. vol. 11, no.3. http://www.osteoporosis.ca/index.php/ci_id/5943/ la_id/1.htm

Osteoporosis Update. Ten-year absolute fracture risk, Fall 2005 vol. 9, no.3, p 4-5. http://www.osteoporosis.ca/local/files/health_ professionals/pdfs/OSTEOFall05edit.pdf

Public Health and Aging: Trends in Aging — United States and Worldwide, National Center for Health Statistics, 2003. http://www.cdc.gov/mmwr/preview/mmwrhtml/mm5206a2.htm

Parkinson Foundation of Canada, 2009. http://www.parkinson.ca/site/c.kgLNIWODKpF/b.5184077/ k.CDD1/What_is_Parkinsons.htm

Serota, A et al. Osteoporosis (Secondary). Emedicine from WebMD, 2010. http://emedicine.medscape.com/article/311449-overview

Siegenthaler W. Differential Diagnosis in Internal Medicine: from Symptom to Diagnosis, Thieme Stuttgart; New York, NY. pg. 369. http://books.google.com

Sutton, R et al. The Intelligent Patient Guide to Osteoporosis, the Intelligent Patient Guide Ltd., First Edition, distributed Gordon Soules Book Publishers Ltd., Vancouver B.C., 2009, Chapter Nine.

Stewart TL et al. "Role of genetic factors in the pathogenesis of osteoporosis." J Endocrinol 2000; 166:235-45.

Theriault, D. "Don't neglect bone health in MS patients." Osteoporosis Update, Spring/Summer 2006 vol.10 no.2, page 5. http://www.osteoporosis.ca/local /files/health_professionals/pdfs/ OsteoSpringSummer05WEB.pdf

Williams LJ et al. "Depression and bone metabolism. A review." Psychotherapy and Psychosomatics. 2009;78(1):16-25. http://content.karger.com/ProdukteDB/produkte.asp?typ=pdf&doi =162297

Prevention and management of osteoporosis: report of a WHO scientific group. WHO technical report series 921, World Health Organization, Geneva, 2003. http://whqlibdoc.who.int/trs/WHO_TRS_921.pdf

Chapter 5
International Osteoporosis Foundation (IOF) www.iof.org

National Institute of Arthritis and Musculoskeletal and Skin Diseases US
www.niams.nih.gov

Ross, P. et al. "Pre-existing fractures and bone mass predict vertebral
fracture incidence in women." *Ann Intern Med*, 1991. 114(11):
p.919-23.

Chapter 6
Spinal Anatomy Animation. Spine Universe.
http://www.spineuniverse.com/anatomy/spinal-anatomy-animation

Chapter 7
Demonstration to get into and out of bed:
http://www.ehow.com/video_4398800_back-pain-tips-getting-out.html

Dodge B. Back Care 101.
http//www.backcare101.com/back-pain-log-rolling

Duragesic® (fentanyl transdermal system) CII. www.duragesic.com
(find more info at: www.webmd.com/pain-management/news
/20080213/ fentanyl-pain-patch-recalled)

Moving safely.
http://www.nof.org/aboutosteoporosis/movingsafely/moving
or an online

Proper pillow placement for sleeping positions.
www.hubpages.com/hub/pillow_placement

Protect your back when getting out of bed.
http://backandneck.about.com/od/activitiesofdailyliving/ss/
backapainsleep1.htm

Chapter 8
After the vertebral fracture, NIH Osteoporosis and Related Bone
Diseases National Resource Centre, US, 1998.
www.niams.nih.gov/Health_Info/Bone/default.asp

Boqing C. et al. Epidural steroid injections, eMedicine, WebMD,
Feb. 2009. http://emedicine.medscape.com/article/325733-overview

Cluett J. Epidural Steroid, About.com, May 2004.
http://orthopedics.about.com/cs/backpain/a/epiduralsteroid.htm

References & Resources

Eidelson SG. Back Pain Treatment Options, SpineUniverse, 2005.
http://www.spineuniverse.com/dispaly article.php/articel1477.html

Hileman C. et al. Calcitonin may be helpful in treating bone pain from
acute osteoporotic vertebral compression fractures, 2004.
http://sfghdean.ucsf.edu/barnett/EBM/CATs/0405HilemanPain.pdf

Mazanec D. et al. "Vertebral Compression fractures: manage
aggressively to prevent sequelae." Cleveland Clinic J Med 2003;
vol.70, no.2, p 154.

Melzack R. The Gate Control Theory of Pain, Canadians for Health
Research. http://www.chrcrm.org/en/node/717

Miacalcin. http://www.pharma.us.novartis.com/product/pi/pdf/
miacalcin_nasal.pdf
http://www.pharma.us.novartis.com/product/pi/pdf/miacalcin_
injection.pdf

Morelli V. "Battling pain with a pill." St. Petersburg Times,1992, p.12.

Solomon D. et al. Cardiovascular risk and NSAID use, Arthritis
Foundation. http://www.arthritis.org.

Wallis C. "The Right and Wrong Way to Treat Pain." Time magazine,
Feb.28, 2005, p. 34 and 36.

What is Chronic Pain? SpineUniverse.
www.spineuniverse.com/displayarticel.php/article1706.html

Wei N. Lumbar epidural steroid injection, arthritis-treatment-
and-relief.com, 2004. http://www.arthritis-treatment-and-relief.com/
lumbar-epidural-steroid-injection.html

White A. III, Your Aching Back, Simon and Schuster/ Fireside, N.Y.,
1990 p. 89-91.

Chapter 9

Acupuncture: an introduction, National Centre for Complimentary and
Alternative Medicine, 2007. http://n:ccam.nih.gov/health/acupuncture.

Acupuncture, National Centre for Complimentary and Alternative
medicine U.S.
http://nccam.nih.gov/health/acupuncture/

Canadian Federation of Clinical Hypnosis. www.clinicalhypnosis.ca

Hochschuler S. Ahh... Ice massage therapy for back pain relief, 2006. http://www.spine-health.com/treatment/heat-therapy-cold-therapy/ahhice-massage-therapy-back-pain-relief.

Mooney V. Benefits of heat therapy for lower back pain, 2003. http://www.spine-health.com/treatment/heat-therapy-cold-therapy/benefits-heat-therapy-lower-back-pain.

Mueller B. Massage therapy for lower back pain, 2002. http://www.spine-health.com/wellness/massage-therapy/massage-therapy-lower-back-pain

National Guild of hypnotists. http://www.ngh.net/

Reiki, National Centre for Complimentary and Alternative medicine U.S. http://nccam.nih.gov/health/reiki/

Rostocki, S. Hypnosis for back pain, cure-back-pain.org, 2009. http://www.cure-back-pain.org/hypnosis-for-back-pain.html

Taylor T. Sacred Space, Reiki. http://www.asacredspace.ca/treatments/

What is reiki? The International Centre for Reiki Training. http://www.reiki.org/faq/whatisreiki.html

White, Augustus, A., III, *Your Aching Back*, Simon and Schuster, Fireside, N.Y., 1990 p. 94.

Chapter 10
American Occupational Therapy Association, Inc. http://www.aota.org.

American Osteopathic Association. http://www.osteopathic.org.

American Physical Therapy Association. http://apta.org.

Canadian Association of Occupational Therapists. http://www.caot.ca.

Canada's Occupational Resource Site. Http:// www.otworks.ca.

Canadian Physiotherapy Association. http://thesehands.ca.

Davis D et al. Transcutaneous electrical nerve stimulation (TENS), 2000. http://www.spineuniverse.com/treatments/physical-therapy/transcutaneous-electrical-nerve-stimulation-tens.

Mitchel S et al. Physiotherapy Guidelines for the Management of Osteoporosis, Chartered Society of Physiotherapy, U.K., 2001. http://www.csp.org.uk/uploads/documents/OSTEOgl.pdf.

Muscle Exercise with Electronic Muscle Stimulation (EMS) TS-131, Mylon Tech Health Technologies Inc, 2003.

Ontario Association of Osteopathic Manual Practioners. http://www.osteopathyontario.com.

Osteopathic College. http://www.osteopathiccollege.com

Smits-Engelsman B et al. Clinical practice guidelines for physical therapy in patients with osteoporosis, Royal Dutch Society for Physical Therapy, KNGF, 2003. https://www.cebp.nl/media/m13.pdf.

Chapter 11

Calf stretch, see VHI lower leg-5 gastroc. http://www.mrfitnessinc.com/fitness/Stretching/Male/Legs.pdf

John Hopkins, Health Alerts, Exercises to help Build Bone Strength and Help Prevent Osteoporosis. http://www.johnshopkinshealthalerts.com/reports/ back_pain_ osteoporosis/2022-1.html

Leg extensions- strengthening the hamstring. http://www.ehow.com/video_ 2360078_ strengthen- hamstring-exercises-seniors.html.

Lloyd L. Fit Society, American College of Sports Medicine. http://www.acsm.org/ AM/Template.cfm?Section=Home_Page& TEMPLATE=/CM/ContentDisplay.cfm&CONTENTID=1258

Low back stretch. No. 12. http://mikesbikes.com/articles/stretching-after-you-ride-pg240.htm.

Mid-back exercise with resistance band, American Council of Exercise, see no.7. http://www.acefitness.org/getfit/rubrbndwkout.pdf.

Mayo Clinic, Exercising with osteoporosis: stay active the safe way, Oct. 3, 2008. Wayhttp://www.mayoclinic.com/health/osteoporosis/HQ00643/ NSECTIONGROUP=2

Morisset Catherine, Life Wellness Coach. Yoga, Fitness & Medical Exercise, phone: 613-737-3428. www.catherinemorisset.com.

Neck stretch. http://video.about.com/exercise/Neck-Stretches.htm.

Neutral spine video. http://www.clearlyhealth.com/videos/osteoporosis/diet_and_exercise/neutral_spine.

Shoulder shrug. http://mikesbikes.com/articles/stretching-after-you-ride-pg240.htm.

Sitting knee extension. http://www.ehow.com/video_2360077_knee-strengthen-thigh-muscles-seniors.html.

Standing stretch, see Arms 1- biceps, Nov. 2009. http://www.leanandgreencoaching.com/uploads/Stretch__Strengthen.pdf.

Straight leg-raise–hamstring stretch. http://mikesbikes.com/articles/stretching-after-you-ride-pg240.htm.

Strong Core, All Spirit Fitness. http://www.allspiritfitness.com/library/QandA/qa_core.shtml.

What are your core muscles? http://beebleblog.com/2007/10/19/what-are-your-core-muscles.

Wall push-up. http://www.5min.com/Video/Wall-Push-Up-18630700.

Chapter 12

Bicycle. http://www.giant-bicycles.com/en-US/bikes/lifestyle/600/28459.

Bone Basics, Moving Safely, National Osteoporosis Foundation. http://www.nof.org/osteoporosis/Guidelines_for_Safe_Movement.pdf.

Check list for a pain-free home office from relax the back. http://www.spineuniverse.com/displayarticle.php/article703.html.

How to sit at a computer. http://www.wikihow.com/sit-at-a-computer.

Influence of yard work & weight training on bone mineral density among older US women, the department of health science, the university of Arkansas. http://www.informaworld.com/smpp/content~content =a904268656&db=all.

Martin, Margaret. http://www.melioguide.com.

Nordic Walking Video. http://www.youtube.com/watch?v=ZKTufkzpo8E.

Tips for Daily Living. http://www.osteoporosis.ca.

Tone Your Bones. http://www.toneyourbones.org.

Chapter 13
Spine University.
http://www.spineuniverse.com/treatments/bracing/spinal-bracing.

Video on back brace.
http://www.spineuniverse.com/treatments/bracing/back-neck-braces-animation.

Chapter 14
Canadian Radiologists who perform vertebroplasty. Canadian Family Physician, Clinical Review, Back Stab, Percutaneous Vertebroplasty for severe back pain, Vol. 53, July. 2007 http://www.cfp.ca/cgi/content/full/53/7/1169.

Complications Associated with the Use of Bone Cements in Vertebroplasty and Kyphoplasty, Health Canada. http://www.hc-sc.gc.ca/dhp-mps/medeff/ advisories-avis/prof/_2007 /bone_cement-ciment_acrylique_nth-aah_2-eng.php.

Efficacy and Safety of Balloon Kyphoplasty, Webinar, Va Meirhaeghe J. AZ Sint-Jan Hospital, Brugg, Oostende, Belgium. http:// kyphon.com.

Johnell O et al. "An estimate of the worldwide prevalence and disability associated with osteoporotic fractures." *Osteoporosis Int.* 2006;17(12):1726-1733.

Kyphoplasty procedure demonstration video, John Finkenberg, M.D., (Note: Kyphon, the company who makes the kyphoplasty device, was bought by Medtronic in 2007). http://kyphon.com.

Kyphoplasty, Spine Institute of New York Beth Israel Medical Centre, video. http://www.spineinstituteny.com/treatments/kyphoplasty.html.

Ng HoiKee. "Kyphoplasty for osteoporotic vertebral compression fractures." *JAAPA* July 2008. http://www.jaapa.com/kyphoplasty-for-osteoporotic-vertebral-compression-fractures/article/124081.

Vertebroplasty and kyphoplasty.
http://www.radiologyinfo.org/en/info.cfm?pg=vertebro.

Vertebroplasty video. http://www.radiologyinfo.org/en/photocat/gallery3.
cfm?image= VertebroMoviePL.jpg&pg=vertebro.

Weinstein J. "Balancing Science and Informed Choice in Decisions
about Vertebroplasty." *N Engl J Med* ; August 2009.

Chapter 15
Beck L. *Leslie Beck's Nutrition Guide for Women, Managing Your Health
with Diet, Vitamins, Minerals and Herbs*, Toronto, Prentice Hall
Canada, 2001.

Benger M. Ottawa Mindfulness. http://www.ottawamindfulness.ca

Brown HJ. *Life's Little Instruction Book*, Rutledge Hill Press, 1991.

Canada's Food Guide. www.hc-sc.gc.ca/fn-an/food-guide-aliment
/index-eng.php.

Canadian Mental Health Association. http://www.cmha.ca

Craig, Diane. http://www.corporateclassinc.com.

Dombeck M. et al. Self-Soothing Techniques: Relaxation Methods,
Progressive Muscle Relaxation, & Massage, 2006.
http://www.mentalhelp.net/poc/view_doc.php?type=doc&id=9759&
cn=353.

Fredas. Freda Iordanous. http://www.fredas.com.

Hair Junkie by FADS, Ann-Marie Tessier. www.hairjunkie.ca

Image Essentials, Ottawa, Ontario, Canada, Pat Armstrong.
www.imageessentials.ca

Maté G. *When the Body Says No: the cost of hidden stress*,
Alfred A. Knopf, Canada, 2003.

Mental Health America http://www.nmha.org.

Natural healing for depression. http://www.healdepression.com/
werbach.htm.

Robbins A. Personal Power® and Get The Edge® CDs.

Ross, J. The Mood Cure, New York, Penguin, 2002.

Shepherds Fashion Accessories. Ottawa, Ontario, Canada.
(owner: Marlene Shepherd). http://www.shepherdsfashions.com.

Style wise: a fashion guide for women with osteoporosis. National Osteoporosis Foundation. www.nof.org/patientinfo/fashion_tips.htm.

The Depression Centre. http://depressioncentre.net.

Volunteers. http://www.nationalservice.gov/about/volunteering/benefits.asp.

White A. III, *Your Aching Back, A Doctor's Guide to Relief*, Simon and Schuster, New York, 1983.

Chapter 16
American Heart Association. Shaking the Salt Habit. July 2010.http://www.heart.org

Armas L et al. "Vitamin D_2 is much less effective than vitamin D_3 in humans." The *JCEM*; 2004, Vol. 89, No. 11 5387-5391. http://www.jcem.endojournals.org/cgi/content/full/89/11/5387

B.C. Dairy Foundation. bcdairyfoundation.ca

Beck L. *Leslie Beck's Nutrition Guide for Women: Managing Your Health with Diet, Vitamins, Minerals and Herbs*, Toronto, Prentice Hall Canada, 2001, p viii, 183.

Dairy Nutrition.www.dairynutrition.ca/ nutrients-in-milk-products/calcium/ calcium-and-bioavailability.

Dietary Sodium, Heart disease and stroke. Heart and Stroke Foundation Canada. http://www.heartandstroke.com.

Dietary Trends, American. http://www.faqs.org/nutrition/Diab-Em/ Dietary-Trends-American.html

Dieticians of Canada. http://www.dietitians.ca

Feskanich, D. et al. "Vitamin K intake and hip fractures in women: A prospective study." *Am J Clin Nutr* 1999; 69(1):74-79.

Grey-MacDonald K et al. "Food habits of Canadians: Reduction of fat intake over a generation." *Can J Public Health*, Sept-Oct 2000; 91(5):381-385.

Health Canada, *Eating Well with Canada's Food Guide*, 2007. www.hc-sc.gc.ca/fn-an/food-guide-aliment/basics-base/ quantit-eng.php)

Health Canada, Food and Nutrition, Dietary Reference Intakes, 2006. www.hc-sc.gc.ca/fn-an/nutrition/reference/table/ref_vitam_ tbl-eng.php.

Health Canada, Natural Health Products. www.hc-sc.gc.ca/dhp-mps/prodnatur/index-eng.php

National Institute of Health, Office of Dietary Supplements. ods.od.nih.gov/factsheets/zinc.asp.

Rao et al. Lycopene: Its role in human health and disease, AGROFood Industry hi-tech, July/August 2003. http://www.lycored.com/web/ articles/lycopene_its.pdf.

Person L. Vitamin K: "ask the expert" column. The Pearson Institute for Nutrition. http://www.lizpearson.com/liz_books.php?id=60

The Worlds Healthiest Foods, The George Mateljan Foundation. www.whfoods.com/genpage.php?tname=foodspice&dbid=146

Taylor N. Green Tea: The Natural Secret for a Healthier Life. http://about.com.

Vitamin D: a key factor in good calcium absorption, July 2010. Osteoporosis Canada. http://www.osteoporosis.ca/index.php/ci_id/5536/la_id/1.htm

Vitamin Supplement Canada. http://vitaminsupplementcanada.com.

Weaver C et al. "Choices for achieving adequate dietary calcium with a vegetarian diet." *Am J Clin Nutri*, Vol. 70, No. 3, 543S-548S, September 1999. http://www.ajcn.org/cgi/content/abstract/70/3/543S.

Wong RWK et al. Effect of quercetin on preosteoblasts and bone defects. *Open Orthop J.* 2008; 2:27. http://www.ncbi.nlm.nih.gov/pmc/articles/PMC2685048.

Chapter 17

General

2010 Clinical Practice Guidelines, for the Diagnosis and Management of Osteoporosis in Canada, CMAJ, Oct. 12, 2010. http://www.cmaj.ca/home/review.dtl or http://www.osteoporosis.ca.

References & Resources

McIlwain H et al. *Reversing Osteopenia, the definitive guide to recognizing and treating early bone loss in women of all ages.* Henry Holt and Company, LLC, NY, 2004; p107.

Osteoporosis Drug Coverage in Canada. *Osteoporosis Update* Winter 2010 vol 14 no. 1 p. 9.
http://www.osteoporosis.ca/index.php/ci_id/5943/la_id/1.htm.

Rona, Z. Bone Density Drugs And the Best Natural Alternatives for Osteoporosis, Vitality, May 2009. Number of people who take BPs-30 million. http://www.vitalitymagazine.com/may09_pg32feat

Watts, NB. Clinical Utility of Biomechanical Markers of Bone Remodeling, Clinical Chemistry, 5:1359-1368,1999.
http://www.clinchem.org/cgi/content/full/45/8/1359.

Calcitonin

Chesnut CH, et. al. "A randomized trial of nasal spray salmon calcitonin in postmenopausal women with established osteoporosis: the Prevent Recurrence of Osteoporotic Fractures (PROOF) study." *Am J Med* 2000;109:267-276.

Cranney A, et. al. "Meta-analysis of calcitonin for the treatment of postmenopausal osteoporosis." Endocrine Reviews 2000, 23 (4): 540-551. http://edrv.endojournals.org/cgi/content/full/23/4/540

Cranney A et al. *Making Choices: Osteoporosis Treatment Options, A Decision Aid for Women with Osteoporosis Considering Treatment Options to Prevent Further Bone Loss and Fractures,* 2002. Copies available in hard copy: call 613-761-4395. Ottawa Hospital Research Institute, 725 Parkdale Ave. Ottawa Ontario, K1Y 4E9.

"Management of osteoporosis in postmenopausal women: 2010 position statement of The North American Menopause Society." *Menopause: The Journal of The North American Menopause Society,* Vol. 17, No. 1, pp. 23-24.
http://www.menopause.org/PSosteo10.pdf.

Miacalcin® (calcitonin-salmon) nasal spray, prescribing information, Novartis.

http://www.pharma.us.novartis.com/product/pi/pdf/miacalcin_nasal.pdf
Product Monograph, Calcimar® Solution (Synthetic Calcitonin-Salmon) sanofi-aventis Canada Inc., May 9, 2006.

Osteonecrosis of the Jaw

BC Cancer Agency Care & Research, Bisphosphonates & Osteonecrosis of the Jaw, Jan. 2008. http://www.bccancer.bc.ca/NR/rdonlyres/ 041F34BF-E05B-4459-A3A7-2428903C6678/27177/ Bisphosphonates and Osteonecrosis of the JawPhysician.pdf.

Khan A et al. "Canadian Consensus Practice Guidelines for Bisphosphonate Associated Osteonecrosis of the Jaw." *J Rheumatol*, 2008; 35:7:1391-1397, Guidelines developed for medical and dental practitioners as well as for related specialists. http://www.jrheum.com/subscribers/08/07/1391.html.

National Osteoporosis Foundation, NOF, Osteonecrosis of the Jaw, June 14, 2006. www.nof.org/patientinfo/osteonecrosis.htm

Osteoporosis Canada, statements on ONJ, June 2007 & Jan. 2008. http://www.osteoporosis.ca/index.php?ci_id=8661&la_id=1.

The Bone and Cancer Foundation New York. http://www.boneandcancerfoundation.org/pdfs/osteonecrosis.pdf

Woo S et al."Systematic review: bisphosphonates and osteonecrosis of the jaw." *Ann Intern Med.* 2006 May 16;144(10):753-61. http://www.ncbi.nlm.nih.gov/pubmed/16702591.

Teriparatide

Neer RM et al. "Effect of parathyroid hormone (1-34) on fractures and bone mineral density in postmenopausal women with osteoporosis." *N Eng J Med* 2001, May 10;344(19):1434-1441.

Parathyroid Hormone (PTH). Osteoporosis Canada. http://www.osteoporosis.ca/index.php/ci_id/5520/la_id/1.htm

Selective Estrogen Receptor Modulators (SERMs)

Barett-Connor et al. "Effects of raloxifene on cardiovascular events and breast cancer in postmenopausal women." *N Eng J Med* 2006;355:125-37. http://content.nejm.org/cgi/content/full/355/2/125.

Canadian Encyclopedia. http://www.canadianencyclopedia.ca/ index.cfm?PgNm=TCE&Params=M1ARTM0011471.

References & Resources

Cranney AB at al. *Making Choices: Osteoporosis Treatment Options, A Decision Aid for Women with Osteoporosis Considering Treatment Options to Prevent Further Bone Loss and Fractures*, 2002.

Cranney, AB et al. "Meta-analysis of raloxifene for the prevention and treatment of postmenopausal osteoporosis." *Endocr Rev* 23(4): 524-528, 2002.
http://edrv.endojournals.org/cgi/content/full/23/4/524?ijkey
=6e31b186008cb2786bf0892de83cfa0584f2b870&keytype2
=tf_ipsecsha.

Cummings SR et al. "The effect of raloxifene on risk of breast cancer in postmenopausal women: results from the MORE randomized trial. Multiple Outcomes of Raloxifene Evaluation (MORE)." JAMA 1999; 28 (23) 2189-97.

Ettinger, B et al. "Reduction of Vertebral Fracture Risk in Postmenopausal Women With Osteoporosis Treated With Raloxifene, Results From a 3-Year Randomized Clinical Trial." JAMA. 1999; 282:637-645.
http://jama.ama-assn.org/cgi/content/abstract/282/7/637.

Strontium Ranelate

Meunier J et al. "The effects of strontium ranelate on the risk of vertebral fracture in women with postmenopausal osteoporosis." *N Eng J Med* 2004;350:459-468.
http://content.nejm.org/cgi/content/abstract/350/5/459.

Reginster JY et al. "Strontium ranelate reduces the risk of nonvertebral fractures in postmenopausal women with osteoporosis: treatment of peripheral osteoporosis (TROPOS) study." J Clin Endocrinol Metab Vol. 90, No. 5 2816-2822, 2005. http://jcem.endojournals.org/cgi/content/abstract/90/5/2816

Roux C et al. "Strontium ranelate reduces the risk of vertebral fracture in young postmenopausal women with severe osteoporosis." *Annals of Rheumatic Disease,* 2008 Dec;67(12):1736-8.
http://www.ncbi.nlm.nih.gov/pubmed/18713788

Strontium ranelate consumer medicine information, national prescribing service limited (NPS), the non-profit organization for quality use of medicines funded by the Australian Government Department of Health & Aging.
http://www.nps.org.au/__data/assets/pdf_file/0003/26796/secproto.pdf

O'Donnell S et al. "Strontium ranelate for preventing and treating postmenopausal osteoporosis." Cochrane Database of Systematic Reviews 2006, Issue 4. Art. No.: CD005326. DOI: 10.1002/14651858.CD005326.pub3

Servier website protelos.com

Strontium

Advanced Orthomolecular Research. http://www.aor.ca/html/products.php

Tibolone

Cummings SR et al. "The effects of tibolone in older postmenopausal women, LIFT trial." *N Eng J Med*, 2008:359:697-708. http://content.nejm.org/cgi/content/short/359/7/697

Robb-Nicholson C. "What's the latest on tibolone, the estrogen alternative?" Harvard Health Publications, Harvard Medical School, April 2004. http://www.health.harvard.edu/newsweek/Whats_the_latest_on_tibolone.htm

Parathyroid Hormone 1-84

"Management of osteoporosis in postmenopausal women: 2010 position statement of The North American Menopause Society." *Menopause*, Vol. 17, No.1, 2010, pg. 44. http://www.menopause.org/PSosteo10.pdf.

Preotact, Parathyroid Hormone website. http:// www.preotact.com

Lasoxifene and Bazedoxifene

Cosman, F et al. "Clinical and mechanistic insights into novel agents in development for osteoporosis." Current Medical Evidence, April 2009.

Kanis JA et al. "Bazedoxifene reduces vertebral and clinical fractures in postmenopausal women at high risk assessed with FRAX®." *Bone,* the Official Journal of the International Bone and Mineral Society 2010; Vol. 44;issue 6: 1049-1054.

Miller PD et al. "Effects of bazedoxifene on BMD and bone turnover in postmenopausal women." *J Bone Miner Res* 2008;23:525-535. http://www3.interscience.wiley.com/journal/123196688/abstract.

References & Resources

Silverman SL et al. Efficacy of bazedoxifene in reducing new vertebral fracture risk in postmenopausal women with osteoporosis." *J Bone Miner Res* 2008;23:1923-1934. http://www3.interscience.wiley.com/journal/123196897/abstract.

Denosumab

Cummings SR et al. for the FREEDOM Trial. Denosumab for prevention of fractures in postmenopausal women with osteoporosis. *N Engl J Med.* 2009; 361(8):756-65. http://content.nejm.org/cgi/content/abstract/361/8/756.

"FDA Panel suggests limits for Amgen's Bone Drug." *The Wall Street Journal*, Aug. 17, 2009. http://online.wsj.com/article/SB125020163968730357.html.

Silverman SL et al. Denosumab in post-menopausal women with low bone mineral density. *N Engl J* Med 2006;354:821-831.

NAMS Position Statement, *Menopause*, Vol. 17, No.1, 2010, pg. 45.

Odanacatib

Odanacatib http://en.wikipedia.org/wiki/Odanacatib.

Odanacatib 2008. http://www.medicalnewstoday.com/articles/121804.php.

Perez-Castrillon JL et al. "Odanacatib, a new drug for the treatment of osteoporosis: review of the results in postmenopausal women." Journal of Osteoporosis, Volume 2010 (2010). http://www.sage-hindawi.com/journals/josteo/2010/401581.html

Drug approval process

Drugs From Research Lab to Pharmacy Shelf, Canadian Pharmacists Association, January 2007.http://www.pharmacists.ca/content/hcp /resource_centre/drug_therapeutic_info/pdf/DrugApprovalProcess.pdf

Licensed natural health products. Health Canada. http://www.hc-sc.gc.ca/dhp-mps/prodnatur/applications/licen-prod/lnhpd-bdpsnh-eng.php

Vibration Therapy

"Age Science Bones, It's time to bone up on your health."
Zoomer Magazine, Nov. 2008, pg. 98-100.

Galileo® Whole Body
Vibration http:// www.galileowholebodyvibration.com.

Juvent Dynamic Motion Therapy®
http://www.juvent.com/dmt/wbv.html.

Power Plate®. http:// www.powerplate.com.

Chapter 18
Chronic Pain Found to Increase Risk of Falls in Older Adults, Science
Daily, Nov. 2009. www.sciencedaily.com

Facts and statistics about osteoporosis and its impact, 2009.
International Osteoporosis Foundation. http://www.iofbonehealth.org.

Fall prevention and seniors, City of Ottawa, Ontario, Canada.
http://ottawa.ca/residents/health/living/injury_prevention/senior
_safety/fallprevention_en.html.

Fall Prevention: 6 tips to prevent falls, Mayo Clinic. July 2010.
http://www. mayoclininc.com.

Fall prevention, National Osteoporosis Foundation. www.nof.org

If you fall or witness a fall, do you know what to do? Public Health
Agency of Canada. http://www.phac-aspc.gc.ca/seniors-aines/
publications/public/injury-blessure/falls-chutes/index-eng.php

Preventing Falls and Related Fractures. NIH Osteoporosis and Related
Bone Diseases, National Resource Centre. Jan.
2009. http://www.niams.nih.gov /Health_Info/Bone/Osteoporosis/
Fracture/prevent_falls.asp.

Seniors' falls can be prevented. HealthLinkBC
http://www.healthlinkbc.ca.

What to do if you fall. http://www.culture.gov.on.ca/seniors /english/
programs/seminars/falls/docs/FallTips.pdf.

Chapter 19

Armstrong P. Image Essentials, Ottawa Day Spa.
   http://www.imageessentials.ca.

Craig D. Corporate Class inc. http:// www.corporateclassinc.com.

Jaglal SB et al. "How are family physicians managing osteoporosis?
   Qualitative study of their experiences and educational needs."
   Can Fam Physician 2003;49:462-468.
   http://www.cfp.ca/cgi/reprint/49/4/462.pdf.

McKercher HG. "Family physicians and osteoporosis, meeting the
   challenge." *Can Fam Physician* 2003;49:405-407.
   http://www.cfp.ca/cgi/reprint/49/4/405.

Taylor, L. "Wilbert Keon at 75: Plenty still to give." *The Ottawa Citizen*,
   May 16, 2010.

PERMISSIONS

Illustration on page 39 from Dempster, DW et al. reprinted with permission from John Wiley and Sons (2010).

Illustration on page 45 reprinted with permission from Eli Lilly Company (2010).

Illustrations on page 65 and 69 reprinted with permission of LifeART image copyright (2010) Wolters Kluwer Health, Inc. - Lippincott Williams & Wilkins. All rights reserved.

Illustration on page 67 reprinted with permission from American Journal of Roentgenology.

Illustration on page 71 reprinted with permission from The Ottawa Sun (2010).

ABOUT THE AUTHOR

Christine Thomas has spent the better part of the past decade speaking out about osteoporosis prevention and management. She is a dynamic speaker who has shared her story of living with osteoporosis with audiences across Canada. She chaired the Ottawa Chapter of Osteoporosis Canada for seven years and founded the Strong Bones Peer Support Group. She wrote *Unbreakable* to share what she learned over the course of recovering from five crippling spinal fractures with other women who have or are at risk for osteoporosis and fractures. Proceeds from sales of *Unbreakable* are donated directly to Osteoporosis Canada.

Christine treasures time with her nine-year-old daughter, Chanel, and her husband, Gerry. Growing up in Montreal as the youngest of four girls, she learned the value of family and the support of three older sisters. Her family and friends rallied around and were a big part of her recovery from fracture. One of her better bone success milestones came when she was strong enough to volunteer at Osteoporosis Canada and her daughter's school, two activities she still enjoys doing today. Her husband and daughter share her love of travel—past trips have included France, Alaska, the Caribbean, and, most recently, a journey through Ireland.

A former senior mediator with the Canada Customs and Revenue Agency, who studied at the universities of Carleton, Queen's, and Harvard, Christine now uses her skills as a passionate advocate of awareness, education, and research on osteoporosis.

To contact author visit www.christinethomas.com

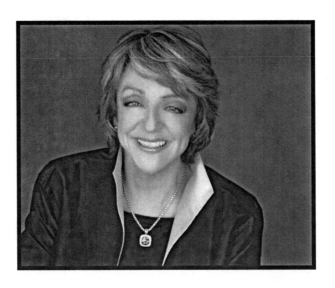

CPSIA information can be obtained at www.ICGtesting.com

226272LV00008B/84/P